Fast To Heal

A 5-Step Guide To Achieving Nutritional PEACE

And Naturally Reversing Chronic Insulin Resistance

Shana Hussin, RDN
Registered Dietitian Nutritionist

Visit:

www.fasttoheal.info

Facebook: Fast To Heal

Facebook Support Group: Fast To Heal Nutrition Support

Instagram: shana.hussin.rdn

Email: shana@fasttoheal.info

Fast To Heal Podcast due out by Summer 2020

Photo Credits: Trisha Weyenberg Photography

ISBN: 9798636298410

DEDICATION

For Paige Emma

Thank you for always believing in me and
being my biggest cheerleader.

Contents

AUTHOR'S NOTE AND DISCLAIMER

The reader should consult their personal physician before beginning any weight loss plan or making changes to their diet. Discuss the material presented in this book with the physician who knows you best before making any changes.

This book is not intended to be a substitute for the professional care of a physician. The reader should regularly consult their physician for all health-related problems and routine care.

INTRODUCTION:

First things first. Take a picture of yourself. I am serious! Do it now, today. I know you may not want to do such a thing, but trust me, you will be glad you did! This is your starting point and you will be happy to see the progress you make. Best to take it of your entire body, and maybe a head shot too. You don't need to share it with anyone just yet. Weeks and months from now, you will be so glad you have documentation of yourself prior to beginning an IF (intermittent fasting) lifestyle and starting the Nutritional PEACE program.

Now weigh yourself. I know this may be painful, but no one needs to know except you. If you can, have someone take your measurements- waist, chest, hips, thighs and upper arms. This will be another way to track progress. It is very powerful and motivating to see inches lost, especially if the scale is not moving as much as you would like or expect.

Before we begin, I need to give you a little background about myself. I graduated with a bachelor's degree in dietetics in 1999, and completed my internship program in dietetics in 2000. I have more or less been practicing in the medical nutrition field ever since. Don't worry, I am not one of those dietitians... you know, the ones who will tell you to never skip breakfast, that you need to eat whole grains in order to be healthy, that you should count all your fat grams. Or that you need to exercise at least an hour every day, that you need to count calories to lose weight, that you can't drink coffee. No, I am not that kind of practitioner, but I admit I used to be!

It has taken me 20 years working with clients in the nutrition field and relentless research, but I have finally discovered the truth about reversing obesity and diseases of insulin resistance. The science I have dug up makes absolute sense, and explains why so many health issues are hormonal issues, not strictly lifestyle issues. In particular obesity, weight gain, metabolic disease, PCOS and type 2 diabetes. I'll admit, for most of my adult life I have not struggled with my weight, I want to be honest about that. But, I had eating issues in high school and college, and I was 2 sizes bigger and 20 pounds heavier in college than I am now, despite being extremely active and avoiding all high fat foods. Most of my immediate family has struggled with weight their entire lives; it was frustrating to be of little to no help to them.

In addition, I have 3 children, and I promise you the baby weight did not just melt away after any of my deliveries! I did not recognize my body postpartum. Let's just say I've done the food journals, excessive exercise and calorie counting several times, and I know how overwhelming it is, especially when calorie reduction stops working. I know how it feels when your clothes are too tight and your muffin top hangs over your pants.

I know what it is like to think about your weight all day long, and how the number on that silly scale determines your mood. I know that sometimes your weight causes you to want to be a hermit in your sweatpants, rather than out enjoying life with others, where you belong. I know...

In all seriousness, I am now at a healthy weight, but I was never somebody who could eat anything I wanted without exercising and restricting certain foods. Ever. I have been exercising like a crazy woman since high school, where I was a 3-sport athlete. I have been active my entire adult life. I have lost track of how many half marathons I have run, and I have trained for and completed 2 full marathons. I strength train regularly. I also taught a wide variety of fitness classes in college and up until I got pregnant with my first child. I tell you this not because I want to impress you, but because I really had to work hard to maintain my weight following the standard nutritional guidelines I was taught by the powers that be, and my own field of expertise.

I did not fuel myself well in high school and college, namely because it was in the 90's when fat was "fattening" and I was afraid to eat many foods and entire food groups. Even though I was athletic and thin in high school, I worried about what I ate all the time. I even became preoccupied with food and spent hours looking through food magazines and recipe books, but I never actually *made* or ate any of them, because the ingredients had "fat" in them.

And everyone knew fat made you fat! If I am being honest, and it is high time for honesty in the food and nutrition world, it was this preoccupation with food that led me to study nutrition and dietetics. I was obsessed with food that I wouldn't allow myself to eat.

During this time of food obsession, I was at my highest weight (other than during my 3 pregnancies) and miserable. I ate very little fat, negligible protein, and was hungry all the time. I was lonely, hungry and tired. Eating with others was not fun as I was so restrictive, and I struggled to find something on any menu I would allow myself to eat. Did I mention I was hungry?

Really hungry?

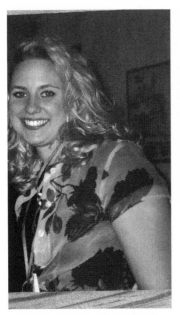 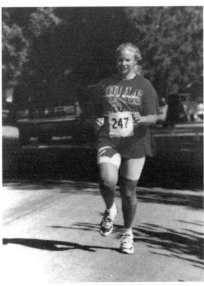

In college (1997-1998), 20 and 21 years old, I weighed 20 pounds more than I do now, and was 2 sizes bigger.

It was around this time that my digestive issues began. I now know why, but it took decades to figure out. I remember in college what I used to eat- a typical day looked something like this... I would limit myself to a banana for breakfast, a large salad at lunch (usually with little meat and low-fat or fat-free dressing- yuck!), and a large bowl of popcorn, or low fat canned soup or another salad for dinner. Sometimes I would have some fat-free sherbet. And, I drank at least 20 ounces of diet coke a day. My 20-year love affair with diet soda began in college, because I hated coffee and got sick of drinking water all the time. But hey, it was calorie and fat free! Who cared about the chemicals? Soda was my "reward" for "being good" and following the obnoxious dietary guidelines. I found plenty of "studies" saying artificial sweeteners were not harmful unless you drank 12+ diet sodas a day, and I was only drinking 1-2. Surely I was fine drinking these vial chemicals!

Here is a confession I have told no one, not even my husband, and I am sure he will be appalled if he reads this. I have lived in Wisconsin my entire life (Go Packers! Go Badgers! Go Brewers!), where beer and alcohol is a big part of our culture, especially at Wisconsin colleges. My freshman year of college I attended the University of Wisconsin-La Crosse, and then transferred to the University of Wisconsin-Stevens Point for the remainder of my undergrad studies. Drinking on weekends was heavy at both colleges. I admit I drank more than my fair share of beers most weekends while enjoying my undergrad years, even though I hated the taste and felt like a truck hit me the next day. It was just what we did. But, my confession is this... I was so hungry and deprived of balanced foods during that time, that when I had a little (or a lot) to drink, I would sometimes eat my roommates' leftover foods out of the garbage while they were asleep.

Now that is completely messed up! I would only feel that much worse the next day because I was ashamed of myself, and, as I will explain, this nighttime eating and drinking was about the worst thing I could have been doing for my health. Then the cycle would begin all over again... I would restrict my food selection all week and drink and eat late on the weekends. I did not feel good about myself. I was a dietetics major with major food issues. Thankfully after I left college I fell into a "normalized" eating pattern and most of my extra weight went bye bye. I was no longer eating and drinking in the wee hours of the night, because by this time I had an adult job that I had to get up early for every day! Also, after I met my now husband, I started to let go of some of my food obsessions and allowed myself to eat some fat and "banned" foods.

I can't believe I just told you that. Now that you know one of my deepest and darkest secrets, let's move on. We are like old friends. No more writing about eating discarded food from the trash! I am thankful I did not contract any major bacterial infection during my binges. And believe me, if you have emotional or binge eating issues, I completely understand where you are coming from. The good news is that my Nutritional PEACE program has fixed emotional and binge eating issues for many people. There is hope!

I didn't eat great in high school either, but I at least ate balanced meals for the most part at dinner, because my mom was brought up eating whole, clean food. We mostly ate at home for dinner, and usually around 5:30 pm. I know I didn't eat enough for my calorie expenditure, however. I was expending a lot of calories playing high school sports, and wasn't eating enough to make up for it. I remember being hungry a lot, but none of the other high school girls ate as much as I wanted to, so neither did I. Admitting I was hungry to other girls, even those who were just as active as I was, seemed out of the question. I know now that restricting my calorie intake decreased my calorie expenditure, and set me up for struggling with my weight and body image.

Hey, side note... now that I am thinking about it, how come it was OK for the athletic boys, or any boy for that matter, to eat 2nd or even 3rds from the high school hot lunch line? And then brag about how much they ate? Oh yeah, because it was socially acceptable and even endorsed! I remember my male friends circling the lunch ladies like vultures for any leftovers that did not get served up that day. It was like winning the lottery for them to eat free hot lunch food that would otherwise be wasted.

Believe me, now that I am old and wise, I am not afraid to eat my fair share in front of anyone, male or female, young or old!

It was in college that my bloating began, almost every day. I remember going home for the weekend and eating certain raw and starchy foods that would bloat me terribly. Even though I knew which foods caused me to feel miserable, I would eat them anyway because they were low in fat and society said they were healthy. I would go back to college Sunday night with a horrible stomachache looking 3-4 months pregnant. My gas was so bad that I sometimes locked myself in my bedroom for the night because I was so stinky and miserable. My roommates just came to know I had gas issues! Thank goodness I had my own room, and my roomies loved me anyway. Plus, all my drinking was extremely inflammatory.

In the years that followed, I tried excluding just about every food, food group, chemical and preservative to alleviate my bloating and pain. I excluded gluten, dairy, artificial sweeteners, sugars and fats. My son was diagnosed with inflammatory bowel disease (ulcerative colitis) in 2016, and together we strictly followed the specific carbohydrate diet (SCD) for 5 months. This diet excludes all grains, sugars, chemicals and additives. I made ALL of our food from scratch and excluded a lot of carbohydrates. This did help and I felt better overall, but I would still get at least minor bloating most days. I also lost weight on this diet and got to the point where I was feeling unhealthy, but I think a lot of the weight loss was due to the constant stress I was under. If you have ever had a chronically ill child, you know what kind of stress that brings. I was maxed out planning, shopping for and preparing everything that went into his mouth. High levels of stress are never good for healing of any kind!

I also tried taking digestive enzymes to help with food digestion, and had specialized testing done to see how I was breaking down my macronutrients (carbohydrates, fats and proteins). In fact, I studied enzymatic therapy extensively in 2019 and became a Certified Digestive Health Professional through the Food Enzyme Institute in Madison, WI. Testing found that I struggle to break down carbohydrates the most, so I took enzymes to help me pre-digest my carbohydrates. This made sense, as it was the high carbohydrate foods that typically lead to my bloating issues. Again, enzymatic therapy did help (about 50%), but I still had minor bloating most days.

My lower abdominal bloating was almost daily for 20+ years until I started intermittent fasting the summer of 2019. It was then that my bloating completely subsided. Now, if I fast for at least 18 hours, I rarely bloat. At all. There were definitely things that helped my bloating, but it was not until I started fasting that my pants fit the same in the evening as they did in the morning. The only time I have minor bloating is if I eat too quickly and don't chew my food well, or I eat way too many carbohydrates, and that is my fault.

I was at a healthy weight when I began IF, but I did lose about 5-6 annoying pounds. Those last stubborn pounds that never want to go away! I also tend to gain a little weight in the summer months. I could never figure out why, but looking back, I likely ate later into the evening and snacked more often because my kids were around. Maybe I was packing on some pounds to survive the harsh Wisconsin winters? All I know is that I did not have to think about my weight at all the summer I started IF, and I haven't had any trouble maintaining my weight since.

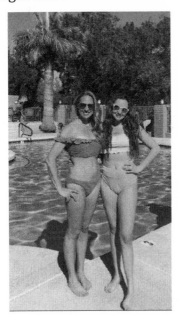 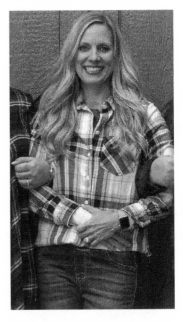

In my mid-forties, 20 pounds lighter, no bloating, no canker sores, more energy, 2019-2020

The other issue that time-restricted eating took care of was my chronic canker sores throughout my mouth, throat and tongue. If you have ever had a canker sore, you know how utterly painful they are. After the birth of my third and youngest child in August 2008, I suffered from canker sores all the time. Never a break. I'm sure my body was depleted and unbalanced, as I had 3 children in 5 years, breastfeeding them all for a year. That didn't leave much time for my body to recover and replenish. Obviously, I also suffered years of sleep deprivation and hormonal changes with 3 small children to raise! I love my husband, but he was not helpful with anything that took place in our home between the hours of 10pm-6am while our children were little. He would say, "I have to work in the morning!" and put a pillow over his head or throw the pillow at me.

But back to the horrible canker sores... Canker sores are open ulcers of the mouth. If you have never had one, consider yourself lucky as each one takes about 2 weeks to heal. I had between 1-5 canker sores in my mouth at all times from 2008-2019. There was never a time I was canker sore free, except for when my dentist prescribed me a special mouth rinse that contained a steroid and antibiotic. This rinse was wonderful, but I hated relying on it for relief, and not knowing what the underlying issue was. So after several months, I discontinued using it. The canker sores came right back. Again, I eliminated every food I thought might be connected, I gave up alcohol for months, I protected my sleep, I took digestive enzymes, I exercised, I tried to manage my stress. Nothing took them away. All of these things helped a little bit and made the healing time a bit less, but I still had at least 1-3 at all times. They were sometimes so painful that I didn't want to talk, smile or eat.

It wasn't until I implemented daily fasts of 16+ hours that the canker sores went away. I am unsure what the cause was, but my best guess is that it may have been a bacterial or hormonal imbalance and not eating as often calmed this down? Or maybe it was the extra gut and mucosal healing that came in the fasting hours. Maybe a combination. I don't know for sure, but I do know I do not miss those pesky canker sores at all! I will follow IF for the rest of my life if it means keeping those awful ulcers out of my mouth.

Looking back, it now makes perfect sense why I struggled with my weight when I did, knowing what I know now. My bloating was likely a result of an overworked digestive system struggling to keep up with food coming in too often. I was eating and drinking late into the night on weekends. I avoided healthy fat and satiating foods. The fat I did eat was processed. I ate a lot of carbohydrates, many of them processed, and drank diet coke all day.

I now want to introduce you to the Nutritional PEACE program, and how it ties in with all that I have learned and implemented to finally heal my chronic health issues and make weight management effortless.

I will lay out the entire program for you later, but PEACE is an acronym for:

P- Prepare your body for fasting

E- Extend your fasts

A- Alter nutrition as needed

C- Clean, Challenge and Change

E- Ease your mind

It is my hope you find a lifetime of good health.

PART 1: WHAT IS INTERMITTENT FASTING?

There are many, many conflicting recommendations about what to eat, but not much focus is placed on when. As a trained nutrition professional, I even grew confused over all the current "studies", and until recently, struggled with what nutrition recommendations to give my clients. Even more frustrating, a diet that worked well for one client, did not work well for the next. One felt great eating vegan while the next preferred keto. Some ate clean or paleo. Others excluded major food groups or all forms of sugars. Yet others felt good on a carnivore, or all meat diet. I scratched my head and researched all of these diets, trying to understand why some thrived on one while the next felt horrible following the same eating plan.

I heard about intermittent fasting on several podcasts I listened to. At first I disregarded it and rolled my eyes when I heard it referenced. Surely skipping breakfast and not eating all day was unhealthy! Every dietitian and nutrition professional knows this. However, I kept hearing the benefits broadcasted from professionals I had a lot of respect for, so I opened my mind and started doing my own research.

I dabbled in IF a little bit in early 2019, but I admit, if I got really hungry 14-15 hours into my fast, I would cave and eat. I have been eating breakfast almost immediately after rising every day my entire life, and everyone knows it is the most important meal of the day! I was one of those kids who ate a bowl of cereal or something similar as soon as I got up. As a child and teenager, I woke early and could never sleep late (this is a blessing and a curse). Even in college, after staying up into the wee hours of the morning, I could only sleep for a few hours after finally going to bed.

Naturally, I have been eating breakfast early my entire existence.

In a nutshell, fasting is basically defined as any time you are not eating. Many health professionals refer to intermittent fasting as time restricted eating, or use these terms interchangeably. Technically, fasting is defined as periods of time, often long periods, when you are not eating. Some fasts are short and some are extended. Time restricted eating is consuming calories only in a set timeframe, such as from the hours of 12pm-6pm. They are very similar, but some argue the terms should not overlap.

For the purposes of this book, I will refer to the periods of time we are not eating as intermittent fasting, but you can think of it as time restricted eating if that makes more sense to you.

Gradually pushing back the time I ate breakfast in the morning worked well for me. It was challenging for me to jump right in and immediately fast 18-20 hours, because I typically wake between 5-6 am, and waiting until somewhere between 12-2 pm to break my fast seemed like an eternity. Some will agree that fasting and blood sugar control can be more challenging for women, as they do not have as much muscle mass or glycogen storage in the liver, as men. Also, because women have higher levels if estrogen, this can sometimes play a role in their ability to fast long time periods.

I am also a distance runner and the thought of running in a fasted state scared me. Early on, the mornings before I left for a run, I would eat a little something the first several weeks I tried IF. So really, I was probably only intermittent fasting 2-3 times per week for 12-15 hours when I first tried to adapt this strategy. Now, I am able to run early mornings in a fasted state, and I actually feel more energized. I like the feeling of no food in my system to bog me down and cramp me up. After I run, I typically wait several hours before opening my eating window. I have been sweetly surprised at how good I feel following a run, and don't feel the need to immediately fuel. I also strength train 1-2 times per week in a fasted state. This transition took some time, as my body was so used to having constant carbohydrates to use for fuel. Now, because I fast for more hours than I feast, my body has learned to use fat for fuel, and making the conversion from carbohydrate stores to fat stores while I exercise is much more efficient.

While researching the benefits of fasting more extensively for a weight loss program I developed in 2019, I stumbled upon *The Obesity Code* by Dr. Jason Fung. Dr. Fung is a nephrologist (kidney specialist), and his book blew my mind. It made so much sense! I remember sitting in my office with my jaw dropped, soaking in all his concepts and research. I grew rather obsessed with his work. I listened to his podcasts, studied his blog and website, and watched his YouTube videos.

After reading his book and following his work, I achieved a level of understanding regarding weight gain/loss that I never had before in all my years of work in the nutrition and medical field. In fact, I am angry this information was not explained to me earlier in my career. I could have helped so many more people!

The problem is, I was taught many concepts that are wrong, and most medical professionals are. Believe me, most practitioners want to help their patients, but they are not given the correct tools to guide them, especially when it comes to obesity, diabetes, PCOS, and metabolic illness. There are many reasons for this, but let's suffice to say that most if it all comes back to money.

Big Food and big money.

Food companies do not make money on people eating less and fasting, friends! They need you addicted to their fake, cheap food, and they don't care who gets sick from eating it! They want you and all those around you to eat their factory-made food, and eat a lot of it. And get addicted. And then get sick and gain weight. And then eat more.

Nobody makes any money when you eat less, and exclude packaged foods.

Breakfast is the most important meal of the day- for Big Food companies.

Eating in a timed window will simplify your life and provide your body with many benefits. It is really that simple! For example I typically fast 18-22 hours a day and I eat my food within a 2-6 hour window. I try to finish my dinner around 6pm, and then I fast until somewhere between 12-4pm the next day. That is what I feel comfortable with and it works for me.

However, many extend their fasts, or eat one meal a day (OMAD). I try to do at least 1-2, 24-hour fasts a week, so I maybe eat a small snack and for sure dinner that day.

Again, my primary goal is not weight loss and I don't have any major health issues, so you need to experiment with different eating windows, and then decide what works for you. If you have been overweight or obese for many years or even decades or you are trying to reverse diabetes, your eating windows may need to be shorter, and you would likely benefit from longer fasts (more on that later).

When I first started fasting, I would only fast for about 15-16 hours, which would be a 15:9 or 16:8 pattern. I slowly pushed back the time that I would break my fast each day over several weeks, until I was omitting breakfast all together and my first meal would be lunch around noon. I love fasting the days I work with clients as my mind is occupied. The days I am not as physically active, fasting feels easier for me. I would suggest fasting for a minimum of 16 hours a day, as this is where some fat burning typically starts to take hold. Fasting even another 2-4 hours beyond that brings many more benefits.

Contrary to what we have been taught, it is not necessary to eat the moment we wake up. Our body naturally stimulates us as we wake. Each morning, counter-regulatory hormones (cortisol, epinephrine and adrenaline) are released. These signals tell your liver to make new glucose and wake you up. All these hormones release glucose into the blood for quick energy. This phenomenon is called the dawn effect. Our bodies are gearing up for action in the morning, not for eating. Morning hunger is a learned pattern that takes place over decades. There is no reason to refuel with donuts, sugary cereal and giant bagels as soon as you get up!

A good starting point is to not eat after dinner. This concept was easy for me because I had long eliminated evening snacking. Believe me, there had been many years of eating a little ice cream or a piece of fruit, or some popcorn before bed. I figured out I slept much better when I didn't eat several hours before bed. I can't tell you how many times I ate ice cream shortly before bed, only to wish I hadn't because it always gave me a stomachache! *Tip: the best way to avoid ice cream before bed is not to have it in your house. Ha!*

Do not eat or drink any calories at least 3 hours before bed. Follow this guideline as much as possible. My goal is not to take away all your favorite foods, but we do need to establish guidelines for success with IF, weight loss and reversing insulin resistance. Not eating or drinking any calories at least 3 hours before bed may be a challenge for you, but it is necessary most of the time. After all, you are fasting! This includes beer and alcohol. Anything with calories is going to break your fast. Sorry!

The good news is, you can include just about any food, on occasion, in your eating window, and eating windows can be flexible from day to day! For example, if you go out to dinner with friends on a weekend and eat dinner or have drinks later than usual, you can fast longer the next day. I would not recommend overdoing alcohol, as it can mess up your electrolyte balance and make it very challenging to fast the next day, especially if you are drinking well into the evening. Anyone who has ever had a hangover knows the next day you crave greasy, salty foods that are refined, and a lot of them. Fasting is about the last thing you want to do.

If there is a day or two during the week that you really want to enjoy breakfast with someone or for a special occasion, do it! You can fast longer the next day, or shorten up your eating window and have an earlier lunch or dinner. This is a lifestyle and you need to make it work for you.

Some people do very well with one meal a day (OMAD). I practice this about once a week. It takes some getting used to, but it really simplifies your day! No breakfast preparation, no packing lunch, no cleaning up, less planning, and more money saved. I don't see a downside! This is easier for me while I am away from home, as I don't have access to my pantry. Practice this concept while at work as co-workers generally frown upon you stealing and eating their food.

Of course there are exceptions, but in general, the longer you fast, the greater the benefits, although I wouldn't recommend fasting beyond 3-5 days without medical supervision. For those wanting support during extended fasts, you can work with me individually.

Others like to rotate their fasting days into a 4:3 or 5:2 pattern. Meaning, they fast for 3 or 2 entire days out of the week, and then eat 2-3 meals on the other 4-5 days, fasting for about 12 hours (mostly while they sleep). For example, you would not eat at all (but of course you would stay hydrated) on Monday, Wednesday, or Friday, but you would eat your normal meals the other 4 days. Both approaches are beneficial, you just need to figure out what works best for you.

The biggest concern those beginning IF seem to have is.... Hunger! Yes, you will be hungry at first; I am not going to lie. If you are eating a lot of processed foods, it may take a little longer to adapt. I still sometimes get hungry during my fasting time, but not nearly as much as I used to. I have learned to ignore it. The whole point of fasting is to not eat, so of course you will be hungry some of the time! You may have more difficulty with hunger if you have been eating frequently throughout the day or are used to eating the moment you get hungry, or eating when you're not hungry at all.

Here is the thing: Hunger comes in waves. If you ignore it, it will go away within a few minutes. It is not persistent. As long as you are feeling good and are not shaky, light-headed or nauseous, ride out the hunger and you will be fine. *IT IS OK TO BE HUNGRY FOR A WHILE!* As a culture, we are so used to eating at the first sign or hunger, or even before. Immediate gratification can be a real detriment to weight control and overall health. Learning to put off hunger requires some mental toughness, but gets easier with time. I find myself feeling very proud when I finish up a fast, and I generally feel great during my fasting period.

Of course, if you are really struggling and feel unwell during a fast, you should break your fast and eat. Your body knows best. You can always pick up where you left off the next day and try a longer fast another time. Remember, intermittent fasting is flexible!

Think of intermittent fasting like you're training to run a marathon. You have to train yourself slowly and gradually to be successful. Know that there will be setbacks and days that you will feel like giving up. When you start marathon training, you can't go and run 20 miles the first week if you have never run before and have been sedentary. You would be terribly sore and would likely not finish your training run. You might even throw up! You might give up training entirely after the first run if you don't let your body slowly acclimate and get used to the new stress you are putting it through.

Fasting is the same. It is a stressor. You can't expect to jump into a 3-day fast successfully if you are used to eating processed foods and sugar every 2-3 hours. You need to have a plan and you need to transition into fasting slowly in order to accomplish your goals.

This is why in the first step of Nutritional PEACE we PREPARE our bodies for fasting. We clean up what we eat and work on extending the time in between our meals. This will ensure better success when you start extending your fasting times.

Humans have been fasting for centuries, and it is the oldest therapy and custom for health improvement known and practiced. Sadly, it has seemingly been forgotten in the American culture over the past generation. Up until the 1970's, people mainly ate 2-3 square meals per day, without snacking in between. They ate dinner (maybe even with a stiff drink) and then quit eating until they went to bed. They did not snack. There were very few obese or overweight people. And guess what? They did not exercise profusely! There were few gyms to go to, maybe a local YMCA. There were nowhere near the fitness options and organized sports that we have now. Do older people ever talk about housewives doing yoga or training for a race in the 1950's and 60's? That would have been cool, but no, they do not!

Exercise trends are increasing in America, s†
and sicker. *What is going on?*

Understanding Hormone Drivers

I practiced in the nutrition field for 20 years before I finally
understood the drivers of obesity, type 2 diabetes, polycystic
ovary syndrome and metabolic illness. I wish I could go back in
time and slap my own face for the recommendations I gave
people early in my career, but I only knew what I was taught.

Insulin is a hormone that is a key player in weight gain.
Hormones are chemical messengers that tell the body to do
something. They are all powerful! There are many regulatory
hormones that intermittent fasting can have an effect on. The
hormones insulin, leptin and ghrelin impact how the body
stores fat, as well as your energy levels. Insulin is a storage
hormone; it signals your body to store fat and glucose (sugar).
First, we fill up all our glycogen (carbohydrate) storage
capacity in our liver and skeletal muscle. We can only store so
much glycogen. A typical adult stores about 1800-2000
calories worth, 400 in the liver and 1600 in the muscles. When
glycogen stores are full, your body has to do something with
the extra calories that are not burned off, and it can convert
everything extra to fat.

It is very important you understand the relationship between
the hormones insulin and glucagon. The hormone glucagon
tells your body to break down stored energy when food is not
present or available. This hormone is high in periods of fasting.
As we have learned, insulin signals your body to store energy
as soon as you eat. Insulin (store energy) and glucagon (release
energy) basically tell your body to do opposite things, when
one is high the other is low. *They cannot both be high at the
same time.*

ple with obesity and diseases of insulin resistance, lin has likely been the dominant hormone for months, ars or decades. If insulin has been dominant, which is the ase for most Americans, it can be healthfully balanced out with eating less carbohydrates, periods of intermittent fasting and extended fasts.

Between meals, as long as we don't snack, our insulin levels will go down and glucagon rises, signaling our liver and fat cells to release their stored energy. The liver and muscle cells will release glycogen (glucose) and the fat cells will release fatty acids. We lose weight if we let our insulin levels stay quiet. The entire idea of intermittent fasting is to allow the insulin levels to go down far enough and for long enough that we burn off our excess sugar, and eventually, fat. Yay!

Understanding the relationship between insulin and glucagon is vitally important to weight control. In today's culture, we live in a toxic world of chemical foods. All processed foods, without exception, increase insulin resistance. Insulin resistance leads to higher and higher insulin to glucagon ratios, and eventually obesity. Having insulin dominant for longer periods than glucagon essentially keeps your body in energy storage mode rather than energy burning mode, regardless of the number of calories you are ingesting.

Why Calorie Deprivation Only Works Short-Term

We need to treat weight gain as the hormonal imbalance that it is. It is not only a calories in vs. calories out problem, as we have been taught for the past 40-50 years. Calorie expenditure is adjusted based on calorie intake, kind of like a thermostat. When you decrease your calorie intake, you will lose weight for a while, but then your calorie expenditure will adjust down to match your calorie intake, and weight loss will plateau. Your body will do everything it can to protect you and maintain homeostasis. It will reduce output when fewer calories are coming in.

Say you typically eat around 2000 calories most days, and decide to decrease your calorie intake to around 1500 to lose weight, as your trusty dietitian recommended. You write down everything you eat and increase your activity. You start to lose about 1-2 pounds per week. Hurray! Life is good!

About 3 months later your weight loss starts to stall. You decrease your calorie intake even further, to around 1200 calories. You spread your food out into small, frequent meals to "keep your metabolism high". You lose a few pounds, but that is all. You know you are not taking in more than 1200 calories because you feverishly journal everything you eat! You increase your activity, but this just makes you hungrier, weaker than you already are. You start getting preoccupied with food, and for a moment consider eating dog food, anything that will satisfy your hunger and cravings!

han·gry

(han-gree) adj.

a state of anger caused by
lack of food; hunger causing
a negative change in
emotional state.

You get hungrier, you feel cold and crabby. You can't live like this and give up. You feel like a complete failure and start eating everything you can shove in your mouth. The weight comes back quickly with a vengeance. You think, what is wrong with me? Why can't I control myself? It's not fair! I have bad genes!

It's not your fault. You have been taught all wrong, and so have the vast majority of health professionals trying to help you. The calorie reduction method is backward and will eventually backfire. Our bodies are designed to conserve body fat at all costs when under periods of calorie reduction. We have been taught to work against our hormones instead of with them.

Think of it like this... Your body will turn its thermostat down if there is not enough energy coming in. If you lost your job and had a hard time paying your energy bill, you would turn your thermostat down from 72 to 65 to save money, correct? Your body does the same thing to conserve energy. Your internal thermostat decreases over time when calorie intake is reduced.

If you keep decreasing your calorie intake, your calorie expenditure will decrease along with it. Your internal thermostat is turned down even further. Calorie reduction will work for about 3-4 months. After that, your calorie expenditure will adjust down to match calorie intake. By this time, most calorie restricting weight loss plans fail, because you can only reduce your calorie intake so far before you become completely miserable, and eat more!

This is why 99% of those who reduce their calorie intake to lose weight will eventually fail.

Obesity and insulin resistance is not a result of lacking resources or willpower; it is a result of a lack of knowledge for understanding the framework of obesity.

By keeping our calories at 0 during a fast, insulin is kept quiet and we can use **our fat reserves for energy** while fasting. Then, by eating until satiated during our eating window, our bodies will keep our metabolic rate normal, as it is provided the nourishment it needs. Because it is using fat stores for energy during the fasting period, metabolic rate does not slow. How awesome is that?

Obviously, if you fast regularly you will lose weight, but more importantly, you will lower your insulin level. Remember, insulin tells the body to store energy. Insulin will be released anytime you eat anything. Not all foods will create the same insulin response, which will be covered later, but any food eaten will stimulate insulin. For example, an avocado (fat) will not stimulate insulin to the same degree as a donut or soda (sugar), but both will stimulate insulin to a certain degree.

By not eating for longer periods of time, your insulin levels are kept quiet, and stored body fat can be accessed. If you're trying to burn body fat there is really nothing better than fasting!

Those who are insulin resistant, which is a very high percentage of people eating a Westernized diet, have a hard time losing weight because there is too much insulin circulating, and the body is constantly told to store energy. After a while, the insulin receptor sites become resistant to the constant insulin, and the extra energy is kept out of the cell, floating around in the bloodstream. This creates excessive sugar in the blood because it is not being let into the cells.

Eventually, prediabetes and type 2 diabetes develops. Extra insulin will only make the problem worse because it will signal the body to force more energy into cells that are already resistant, and a vicious cycle ensues. More insulin, more fat storage, more weight gain.

Fat burning is mostly determined by insulin, which is a nutrient sensor. Your body needs to know whether or not nutrients are coming in, and really only exists in one of two states, fed or fasted. In the fed state insulin is high. When you eat, insulin goes up, signaling the body to go into a fed state and store energy. You will store limited energy as carbohydrate in your liver and muscle tissue. After that, it is stored as fat, and fat storage is unlimited!

If you eat extra protein, more than you need, your body doesn't really have the ability to store much extra protein. There is some extra that circulates in your bloodstream, but after that the excess is converted and stored as glucose. **Sorry, extra protein is not used to bulk up, friends!** If that were true, we could all eat piles of meat and look like bodybuilders. Regular strength training and available growth hormones tell the body to build extra muscle. If your glucose stores are full in your liver and muscle, your body will then convert extra protein into fat in a process called lipogenesis.

To be in a fat burning state, you can't be constantly stimulating insulin. This is why calorie deprivation can be so completely frustrating. At some point you were likely advised to decrease your calories down to 1200-1800, depending on your size, to lose weight. You were told to eat those calories spread out in small, frequent meals in order to "maintain your metabolism". The calorie deprivation will work for a little while, but then you will plateau as your body adjusts its output to match intake. Because you are eating small, frequent meals your insulin is constantly high, signaling your body to store energy coming in. As a result, you continue to gain weight even on lower calories. Maddening!

Once you realize that fat burning is all about hormonal influence, you realize how utterly insane it is to be advised to eat all the time, 5-6 times per day (or more), in order to lose weight!

Remember, *we need insulin* and it is natural to store food energy. It is how humans have survived for millennia. Your body needs to store energy and be able to burn it at a later time. It is the reason why you don't die in your sleep every night, because you are able to use energy stores to keep your brain and body alive. The problem is when our insulin is always high and glucagon is low. These two hormones become out of balance, and then you start storing food energy more than you are breaking it down. The result is weight gain.

If you want to lose weight you need to burn food energy more than you store it. That's what body fat is; stored energy. It is natural to store energy, that's what body fat is designed for. What your body isn't designed for is eating all the time and eating processed, starchy foods constantly. If you keep eating all the time, you will not give your body the opportunity to burn fat. Insulin impedes fat burning. Body fat is either being stored or burned; your body can't do both at the same time.

Fasting is a quick way to lower insulin. By lowering insulin, your body can access stored body fat. If you simply eat low fat and reduce calories, but eat 6-8 times per day, you're stimulating insulin all day, and therefore, keeping your body in the fed state rather than the fasted state. You need to be in the fasted state to burn excess energy. If you can lower your insulin throughout the day and night, you allow your body to burn some of that stored food energy. You either eat new food, or burn stored food.

Eat a cheeseburger now, or don't eat, and burn off that cheeseburger you ate 2 years ago!

If we go even 40 years back, there was very little obesity, type 2 diabetes or heart disease. Why has it exploded? It's because we eat all the time, and we eat foods that heavily stimulate insulin secretion. In the 1970's snacking was frowned upon, people mostly ate homemade foods without chemicals, and most people ate 2-3 square meals a day, which left at least 12 hours a day to be in a fasted state. If dinner was around 6pm and breakfast wasn't eaten until 8am, it was a 14 hour fast every day. The fed state and fasted state was balanced.

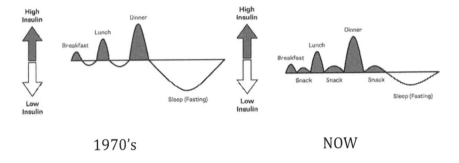

1970's   NOW

Source: *The Obesity Code* by Jason Fung, MD

Americans eat more often than ever before. Insulin is continuously stimulated when meals and snacks are eaten constantly throughout the day, telling our cells to store energy. Glucagon is never allowed to be dominant.

In 2005 the average number of times people ate was 6. More recently, it was found that only 10% of Americans ate about 3.3 times per day or less. That means 90% of the population was eating more than 3 times per day! **The top 10% of people who ate most frequently averaged eating 10.3 times per day**.

In essence, we're staying in a fed state from the minute we get up until the minute we go to bed. And then we wonder why we're so fat as a nation! It's because by eating 10 times a day, you're stimulating insulin 10 times a day, which gives your body instructions to store energy 10 times per day. If you want to lose weight and reverse chronic illness, you can't do that! If you want to lose weight, eat less often so your insulin can fall. Then your glucagon levels will rise, giving your body instructions to start breaking down and burning stored food energy.

Childhood Obesity

The above data gives us a general understanding of why childhood obesity is exploding. First of all, high insulin levels can be inherited from the mother, so if the baby was exposed to high insulin during pregnancy because the mother's insulin was constantly high, that baby already has higher than normal insulin levels at birth.

In addition, we have been completely entrenched with the idea that we should eat all the time. Kids eat breakfast immediately when they get up before school, then they have a snack time at school a few hours later. Then they eat lunch. Then they come home and have another snack after school. Then they have dinner, and likely, another snack before bed. That doesn't even account for all the sugary drinks many children are consuming throughout the day, which also spike insulin. Because they are constantly eating, and usually eating starchy processed foods, their satiety mechanisms are turned off, they are always hungry, and they lose their natural appetite control.

I spent 3 years in our school district substitute teaching, and the vast majority of food served was processed in some way. Sugar is high in almost every processed food, promoting constant insulin secretion. A typical breakfast served at school was a pack of Cheez-its, a sugary yogurt, canned fruit and chocolate milk. No wonder kids act out and have so many chronic issues! They are suffering constant hormonal swings, and eating all the time. And that is only breakfast. I have witnessed children eat an entire sleeve of crackers for a "snack" a few hours after eating breakfast.

Behavior and digestive issues are constant. When I did a long-term substitute teaching job for a 2nd grade classroom, there was one little girl I had to send to the nurses office twice daily for Miralax due to severe constipation. She ate the school breakfast and lunch for free because her family was low-income.

This photo I took of an actual breakfast served while I worked as a long-term substitute teacher for 2nd grade. Other breakfasts were very similar.

So much sugar!

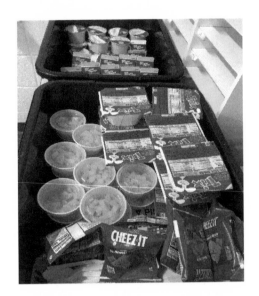

There is a lot of work to do in the area of school nutrition. But that is another book...

Our grandmothers were correct when they told us not to snack in between meals, and to eat less sugar! Nobody counted calories in the 50's and they were fine. No one ate quinoa or veggie burgers in the 60's and they didn't have problems with obesity. Moms were not at the gym doing extensive workouts. People were not keeping food journals and testing ketones.

The key is to not eat all the time!

Last Thoughts on Insulin and Glucagon

Insulin levels begin to drop after you finish eating, and reach their lowest point around 9 hours. Glucagon then begins to rise, peaking around hour 8. After only 9 hours of fasting, we enter into a healthy insulin to glucagon ratio. Ketones (byproducts of fat metabolism) begin to emerge from the liver. Fat cells are released into the bloodstream and excess body fat

storage begins to shrink. Mitochondria becc
fat as energy. Inflammation starts to fall, a'
into an amazing repair and maintenance

After *only 9 hours,* the process of undoing ,
choices from the day before begins and insulin ɾɛ
improves. This is encouraging, except for the fact that ɴ
people eat until they go to bed and again right away in the
morning as soon they get up. Your doctor and dietitian (yes, I
was one of those dietitians, sorry!) tell you to eat often to keep
your metabolism active. As you can see, most Americans
following the schedule of eating all day long never have a
chance to let glucagon levels rise and insulin fall enough to
burn fat. If you eat all day every day, your glucagon is just
beginning to rise 8 hours after you went to bed, and by eating
right away in the morning, insulin rises again and glucagon
falls.

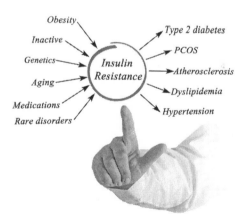

It is critical that you understand that under the influence of
high insulin and low glucagon, **every** macronutrient
(carbohydrate, protein and fat) is eventually converted to fat.
Under the influence of low insulin and high glucagon, **none** of
the macronutrients are directed to be stored as fat.

od news is that you can start to recover and normalize
insulin to glucagon ratio after only 9 hours! *That means
a can start to feel better on this very day!* Keep in mind that if
ou have had elevated insulin for decades, it will take some
time to heal and recover, but it can be done.

Other Hormones to Know About

Thyroid Hormone

Thyroid hormone needs addressing because every cell in our
body has a thyroid receptor site. Let's talk about its function.
TRH (thyrotropin-releasing hormone) is secreted from the
brain, which travels down to the pituitary gland to secrete TSH
(thyroid stimulating hormone). TSH travels down to your
thyroid gland to produce mostly T4. T4 goes out into the body
and gets converted to T3 in the peripheral tissues. It is the free
T3 that is the active form of thyroid hormone. If you are
looking at thyroid function testing, you need to look at all the
parts of the cycle, TSH, T4, T3, free T4, free T3 and reverse T3.
It is also smart to screen for thyroid antibodies, especially in
the case of Hashimoto's disease (low thyroid function due to
autoimmune disease).

Thyroid disease is much more common in women, 5 times
more likely, than men. This is likely due to the effects of
estrogen on the thyroid. If you have estrogen dominance (and
likely insulin resistance), this increases thyroid-binding
globulin (TBG), which is produced in the liver. TBG binds up
your free T4 and free T3.

An interesting fact is that birth control pills also increase TBG,
which can lead to lower thyroid function.

Too much estrogen also inhibits the proteolytic enzymes within the thyroid, and also inhibits the release of T4 from the thyroid gland. Estrogen dominance causes lower thyroid function, the low thyroid function cause more excess estrogen. Another vicious cycle!

Estrogen dominance decreases the conversion of T4 into T3. Without good metabolism of estrogen in the liver, your thyroid can be harmed further. Estrogen dominance is covered at length in the Special Considerations for Women section, but usually insulin resistance is a major player seen in estrogen dominance. If you have known thyroid issues, you should also look at estrogen levels and insulin resistance.

Do we need carbs for a healthy thyroid? Do we need carbs for the conversion of T4 to T3? This topic comes up often when talking about intermittent fasting and thyroid function. It depends. I am not aware of any evidence that carbohydrates are needed to convert T4 to T3, but zinc and selenium do play a strong role. These are minerals found primarily in meat, eggs and shellfish.

In many situations, if low thyroid function is due to estrogen dominance and/or insulin resistance, LESS carbohydrate and intermittent fasting can help heal the hormone imbalances at play.

After pregnancy is a common time to have exacerbations of thyroid issues because estrogen is so high during pregnancy, and the levels come crashing back down within days of childbirth. Excessive estrogen may have been suppressing your thyroid during pregnancy. Sometimes there is a transient increase in thyroid function, and then it will burn out. If you are newly post-partum and have thyroid issues, it is important to have the levels checked often, every 6-8 weeks, to see what is going on with thyroid function.

A low carbohydrate, or even a ketogenic diet can help heal the thyroid gland. **Calorie restriction, however, reduces thyroid function.** Your thyroid gland is related to fertility, so if your thyroid gland senses a decrease in available calories and nutrition, it will try to conserve, reducing metabolic rate. It is important to meet your caloric needs. We have learned this!

In some people, intermittent fasting and the ketogenic diet may decrease free T3 levels. Depending on the health and lifestyle of the individual, slightly lower T3 levels in the active form of the thyroid hormone is not necessarily a bad thing. This is because TSH may increase and thyroid sensitivity improves. If there are no symptoms (being cold, fatigue, weight gain, hair loss) of low thyroid function, there is no reason to think the thyroid is in jeopardy. If the individual is intermittent fasting as a lifestyle, is eating nourishing food and is fat-adapted, slightly lower T3 levels are generally fine in those who are feeling great, have ample energy, are not gaining weight, and are sleeping well.

Those who are eating junk food, excessive processed carbohydrates, and in poor health, intermittent fasting with low free T3 levels can be detrimental.

My advice is to have a discussion with your doctor about your thyroid hormone levels if you think you have thyroid issues, and have all the discussed levels checked prior to beginning any sort of extended fasting. Again, if you are eating nourishing foods and feel well, a lower T3 can be helpful, but if you are eating processed foods and feel unwell, stay in the first 3 Steps of Nutritional PEACE to clean up your diet before challenging yourself with longer fasts.

In theory, if you are in good health and intermittent fasting, slightly lower levels or T3 are likely a result of your body not needing as many thyroid hormones. This is a good thing as it gets more efficient at using available hormones and doesn't have to manufacture as many. If you are constantly eating starchy carbohydrates and in sugar burning mode all the time, you will need more thyroid hormones to balance your body out, putting more pressure on the thyroid.

It is hard to know how you will respond to intermittent fasting until you try it, which is why my program eases you into it. Intermittent fasting can make bigger or smaller impacts on thyroid hormones depending on the person and their overall health and food intake prior to beginning any fasting.

Oftentimes thyroid issues are autoimmune in nature, the majority being Hashimoto's Disease, or hypothyroidism. If there is an autoimmune component to a thyroid issue, most likely the gut is not in a healthy state and needs to be repaired. You may need to really focus on eating nourishing foods and staying with shorter fasts until the gut is repaired before progressing to intermediate or advanced forms of fasting. Refer to the section on Autoimmune Illness to help fix leaky gut.

There is a correlation between lower calorie diets and lower thyroid levels. This makes sense, because if less nutrition is coming in, your body has to dial down its energy expenses, and thus may decrease thyroid hormone. This is why it is so important to take in enough nourishment and eat until you are full in your eating window. We are not calorie restricting! *Don't eat less, eat less often.*

It is important to note that coffee can be detrimental to some. The caffeine in coffee, or any caffeine for that matter, can be over stimulating to the adrenal glands and cause a cortisol rise. This is not helpful as the rise in cortisol may cause a rise in insulin. If you know you have adrenal issues, it is best to drink water, or decaf coffee or tea only during your fast, or exclude caffeine completely.

Those who are struggling with depression or lack of menstrual cycles may have underlying gut issues (leaky gut) and repairing the gut is key to improving symptoms. Your body may have underlying inflammation you are not aware of. Your gut is basically a second brain of sorts, and has far-reaching implications on your hormones. The gut and brain are intricately connected with the gut-brain axis. In addition, 95% of our serotonin (the feel good hormone) is made and stored in our gut. If your gut and microbiome are unhealthy, depression and mental illness can ensue due to lack of serotonin. The Nutritional PEACE program helps heal your gut by improving nutrition and allowing the gut to repair itself while you are implementing fasting periods.

Gut healing won't be completed in one round of fasting; it needs to be part of your life routine. You will slowly rebuild gut lining cells and enterocytes. Fasting also helps to nourish the helpful bacteria in your microbiome and crowd out harmful bacteria. Fasting is a useful tool that can give the body a break and bring overall levels of inflammation down.

As mentioned, I saw this in my own life. I suffered from multiple, excruciatingly painful canker sores in my mouth for 11 years. There was never a time I was without at least one during that time frame. I eliminated so many foods and food groups, praying to find the root cause of my pain. After about 3 months of regular intermittent fasting, they disappeared and have not returned. Balancing out hormone fluctuations and allowing my digestive tract to repair itself while I fasted made all the difference.

Growth Hormone

Insulin and growth hormone are indirectly related. If your insulin is constantly elevated, growth hormone is low. In fact, there is nothing that turns off the secretion of growth hormone more than eating. It is hard to burn fat and build new muscle when growth hormone is low. This is why keeping insulin low increases growth hormone, so when you do eat, you rebuild muscles and tissue that need growth and repair.

When you don't eat and your body starts to go into a fasted state, you will first utilize all your available glucose, what is circulating and then what is stored as glycogen. Then your body may burn some protein sources, but at the same time, it is starting to rev up your fat burning mechanism. We have a ton of fat to burn, but it can be really hard to get at. Even though you do burn some proteins, growth hormone is increasing in a fasted state. When you break your fast and eat, because growth hormone is so much higher than in a fed state, the growth hormone will allow you to put on healthy lean muscle mass.

If you are in a constant state of eating, your body will struggle to go through that complete renovation cycle of breaking down the old proteins that are not working very efficiently.

During a period of at least 15 hours of fasting, cells become more sensitive to hormones. Many people who feel unwell, it is not because they lack certain hormones, it is that their cell receptors can't "hear" the hormones that they do have talking. Taking synthetic or bioidentical hormones, such as estrogen, is very popular and may be helpful for a while. The problem is, if your hormones are normal and the chemical message is not getting into the cell because your body has grown insensitive, you won't feel better.

Intermittent fasting helps make the cell more sensitive to hormones, whether it is insulin, estrogen or thyroid. Weight abnormalities, hair falling out and dry skin are all signs of hormone sensitivity or imbalance. Medications may help blood levels of hormones look normal, but if symptoms persist, hormonal messages are not getting into the cells. There are certain toxins that can prevent the cell from hearing the hormone such as heavy metals and ingested chemicals, but that is a topic for another book! For purposes of this book, it is helpful to know that intermittent fasting improves hormone sensitivity, and your cells better hear chemical messages from hormones.

Keep in mind, if you have significant female hormone, male hormone, or even thyroid issues, take intermittent fasting slowly and follow the steps I lay out in Nutritional PEACE. If you have known leaky gut, work on healing your gut before extending fasts too long or too often. Stay in step 1 until you feel stable and ready to start extending fasts. Take the chemicals and toxins out of foods, and focus on nutrient dense foods to detoxify and heal your gut.

Fasting will impact all of our hormones to a certain degree, as they are all interrelated.

Ketones and the Ketogenic Diet

The "ketogenic" or keto diet dates back about 100 years. In 1921, Dr. Russel Wilder described the term ketogenic diet for a diet that reduces carbohydrates and increases fat. This, in turn, raises ketones in the blood, because fat metabolism uses ketone bodies for fuel. Interestingly, the diet was originally developed as a way to treat children with epilepsy.

The ketogenic diet can be helpful in lowering insulin resistance, leading to weight loss. While I am not against following the keto diet, especially for a shorter time period of around 3-6 months, I am not an advocate of diets that enforce strict guidelines and exclude food groups long-term, or forever. The diet typically recommends a macronutrient ratio of around 75% of calories coming from fat, 20% from protein and only 5% from carbohydrates.

For me, all this counting and monitoring of ketone bodies is far too complex and life altering. Also, the keto community lives in fear of being "knocked out of ketosis". They are fearful of eating carbohydrates and even protein, because protein increases insulin almost as much as carbs. Eating 75% of your diet from fat can be challenging, and I know of some people following the keto diet who exhibit bizarre behaviors, such as eating coconut oil by the tablespoon. Surely this can't be optimal!

With that being said, the keto diet does have its place, especially if only followed for a few to several months, and after that healthy carbohydrates are cycled in. Eating higher amounts of fat can help you convert from a sugar burner to a fat burner and reduce appetite and cravings. For these reasons, it can be very helpful. It can be especially impactful when coupled with intermittent fasting early on if you have a lot of weight to lose or have been insulin resistant a long tome. As medical professionals, we need to realize that some people have a lot of trouble digesting and utilizing carbohydrate, and they need to be minimized at least for a time. Carbohydrates are not inherently "bad", but not all people process them in the same way or capacity.

A very interesting study in dogs shows that protein, in the absence of carbohydrates, leads to a glucagon spike. Remember, glucagon tells your cells to release stored energy and burn it off. Most people following keto are afraid of eating too much protein, but this study suggests that glucagon is even higher after protein is eaten and carbohydrates are absent, than even in a fasted state. In the presence of high glucagon, the body releases fat stores and generates ketones. For this reason, protein need not be feared as long as processed and excessive carbohydrates are kept out of the diet as shown in this study. You can read more about the study here:

https://www.jci.org/articles/view/106706

As previously explained, once you utilize circulating carbohydrates, glycogen stores, and possibly some protein, then your body taps into fat for energy. Your body fat cells are basically released, and triglycerides (fat cells) rise in your bloodstream. Most of your body will utilize triglycerides for energy directly. However, some triglycerides are converted into ketones. An amazing quality of ketones is that they are water-soluble. This means ketones can cross the blood brain barrier and fuel the brain.

Sugar is a really quick fuel to burn. We can convert glucose or sugar into energy very quickly, without the presence of oxygen. There are some benefits to burning sugar for fuel, but it is very metabolically expensive, meaning we produce a lot of waste when we burn glucose. Lactic acid and free radicals are byproducts. Free radicals in large amounts damage tissues in a process called oxidative stress.

Ideally, we want to be able to burn glucose for energy in times when there is not much oxygen present. Running a sprint or intense weight lifting would be examples. When we want to perform at a really high level is when we want to have the ability to burn glucose.

For times when you are not expending intense energy, ketones can be a much more metabolically efficient fuel source. Because they are water soluble, they can easily cross cell membranes and get right into the cell's mitochondria to be used for energy. We produce a lot more cellular energy from a ketone than we do from a molecule of glucose, just not quite as quickly. Ketones produce significantly less oxidative stress and metabolic waste.

If you are insulin resistant, you are better able to burn fats as fuel by taking in less carbohydrate, especially processed starches and sugars. Focus on adding in healthy fats such as avocados, olives, olive oil, grass fed butter, macadamia nuts, coconut oil and coconut products.

Although not required, the ketogenic diet works well with fasting because we get keto and fat adapted, where our body gets used to burning ketones. Our hunger and cravings diminish. If all we do is burn sugar as our primary fuel source, we're rarely, if ever, burning fat.

It is not essential to be in ketosis, but if you want to do a keto diet coupled with intermittent fasting, that is typically a fantastic way to lose weight and improve health. There is a machine called a blood ketone meter where you can measure your blood ketones, which tests beta hydroxybutyrate. You are looking for the state of nutritional ketosis, which is anywhere from 5-6 millimoles. Sometimes people even feel great at levels from .5-1.5 because they are keto adapted, and are able to go long periods without food.

If you hate pricking your finger to get a blood ketone level, you can use a breath ketone meter, which measures acetone in the breath. Acetone is a byproduct of ketone metabolism. You blow into a tube rather than prick your finger.

I'm certain I go in and out of ketosis quite regularly, but I have never tested my ketone levels. It is just not something I want to do, nor do I count my carbohydrate intake, as it doesn't seem like a natural way of eating. I focus on eating whole foods and make sure I eat healthy fats and nutrient dense foods at each meal. I eat very few grains as they make me feel unwell.

Many people do very well following a keto diet plan, but I do not find it necessary to improve health. If you're following keto, you should implement it for 3-6 months, and then start to cycle in some nutrient dense carbohydrates such as beets, carrots, sweet potatoes, potatoes, sprouted grain bread or berries into your eating plan at least weekly or monthly. Every eating plan should be varied after a time period.

Being on a low-carb or very carb-restricted meal plan for many months or years can be compromising for your health. Your body may blunt insulin receptors because it has been without glucose for so long as a fuel. Continuously lowering carbohydrate intake for extended periods of time can cause your body to want to conserve fat. It is definitely a balancing act! This is where nutritional and seasonal variation can be helpful, and cycling in periods of higher, nutrient-dense carbohydrates.

Carbohydrates that raise insulin the most are man-made, no one can argue with this. Carbohydrates created by God in their wholeness with fiber intact have minimal effect on insulin. Breads, cereals, buns, soda, pasta, candy, chips and other processed and refined carbohydrates made in factories, as well as processed oils and fructose, are what make us ill. We can't just label all carbohydrates as bad foods to be avoided. Not all carbohydrates prevent ketosis or the burning of fat.

With that being said, as obese Americans who are insulin resistant, we can no longer eat large amounts of unhealthy carbohydrates. We must first heal our insulin resistance. The treatment is to lower processed carbohydrates as least initially, which will help to lower overall insulin levels, ultimately leading to a reduction in body fat. Decades of insulin resistance first began very early in life with the ingestion of processed American food. The second step is to practice periods of intermittent fasting to keep insulin low, so glucagon can be dominant and fat burning can take place. The longer you can keep your insulin low and glucagon dominant, the more you heal insulin resistance.

Keep in mind there is a subset of people who do very well on a carnivore, or all meat diet. Including organ meats can be very helpful in healing autoimmune illness and inflammation. While I do not recommend everyone follow a carnivore diet, and obviously it goes against what the Academy of Nutrition and Dietetics advocates, there are some who feel very well eating mostly or all meat.

Remember, all diets work, and no diets work!

PART 2: HOW TO GET STARTED

There are many different fasting schedules you can try, there is no one set way that works for everyone. What I do know is that every single person I have worked with has benefitted from intermittent fasting in some way.

First of all, you've got to stop snacking! Snacks are not at all helpful for several different reasons. Snacks are typically convenience foods that are highly processed, and more often than not have a lot of sugar. They are not nourishing if they come in a package. That food is dead! Chances are you are not snacking on salmon; you are snacking on a processed granola bar or a muffin. Even if you are snacking on whole fruits and vegetables, eat them with a full meal to give your insulin a chance to come down in between meals. If you are eating until you are full during your meals and your meals are balanced, you should not need to eat for 4-5 hours between meals if you are eating more than one meal a day.

The next detriments you need to get rid of are sweetened beverages. If you drink them, sweetened beverages are one of the main things ruining your health! Sweetened coffee beverages, juice, soda, sports drinks, energy drinks,

hocolate milk, it's all got to go! This is where
rated and want to stop reading. Trust me... I
20-year love affair with diet soda. It was
up. But you need to decide what is more
.... losing weight and getting healthy, or wasting $3-5
sugar-laden coffee drink every day?

Drinks while fasting suggest a lot of gray areas if you search the murky waters of Google. Some will say diet soda and no calorie drinks are ok during a fast. Some will say butter or coconut oil in your coffee is OK. In my experience, what may be ok for one person is not ok for the next. It's all about insulin stimulation, and anything with sweetness (even artificial) or any sort of calories may stimulate insulin in some people.

I like black and white when it comes to fasting. There are too many variables when it comes to artificial sweeteners and adding things to drinks, and I don't like variables. You can drink water, black coffee or herbal tea that is not sweetened during a fast. Just about anything else may cause an insulin response. Even if there are no calories in your diet soda, your body may sense sweetness and release insulin anyway. Some say diet soda or a small amount of creamer may be ok. I say, why risk it? Save it for your eating window time if you must have it. There is no reason to sabotage your efforts. A fast is a FAST! It may take some time to break yourself of morning habits, but I promise it will be worth it in the end.

Another behavior that needs to go is eating late at night. It's just not a smart thing to do if you are trying to lose weight and become a healthier human. Your body is getting ready to shut down and slow metabolism, so calories you take in at night are likely going to be turned into fat rather than be used for energy. Plus, your body is forced to deal with and digest that food, rather than repair and renew like it is supposed to while you sleep. Another problem with eating late at night is that your hunger tends to peak around 8pm, and there is a bigger insulin effect on the food you eat. You're hungrier so you will eat more, and more insulin is secreted than if you would have eaten that same food earlier in the day.

Start by skipping breakfast. It's an easier meal to skip because eating breakfast is typically done alone or on the fly, and is not as much of a social meal. Also, if you remember, your body releases counter regulatory hormones to wake you up and come out of the sleeping state. Adrenalin increases, activating the sympathetic nervous system. This changes your physiology to wake up. In addition, you have already been fasting while you have been sleeping, so it is an easy way to extend your fast!

Should you weigh yourself?

This is a tricky question because intermittent fasting is not necessarily a quick weight loss plan. Don't get me wrong, some drop weight pretty quickly, especially in the beginning, while others struggle for weeks without dropping a pound. The truth is, there are many processes and a lot of healing going on during fasting times that are not always reflected on the scale. For me, I got rid of daily bloating and chronic canker sores. Losing weight was not my primary goal, but I did lose some belly fat. Hooray!

Take a look at your goals. If one of your primary goals is weight loss, then I think it is a good idea to weigh yourself at least occasionally. With that being said, if you weigh daily, I would encourage you to average your weight out for the week. You can expect to lose about 1-2 pounds a week depending on your fasting schedule. Take your measurements regularly so you can see progress made in inches lost. Look at your weekly averages. Chances are even if your weight loss is not linear day to day, you will still lose weight when you compare weekly averages. Take pictures of yourself often.

Here is an example of how to track and average your daily weights and weekly averages.

Sunday	Mon	Tues	Wed	Thurs	Fri	Sat	Avg
195.1	194.2	194.9	195.2	195.3	195	195.1	**195**
195.9	194.1	194.2	194.2	194.1	193.3	194	**194.3**
194.1	194.4	194.1	192.9	192.4	192.2	193	**193.3**
193.8	193.2	193.8	193.1	193.0	193.9	192.5	**193.3**
193.6	193.2	193	193.4	192.4	191.9	192.8	**192.9**

Sometimes some major or minor healing needs to take place before your body is ready to let go of weight, especially if you have major hormonal imbalances. Give yourself time; don't decide in the first week whether or not this lifestyle will work for you. Try it for a month at the very minimum. Another thing to remember is that toxins are often stored in adipose (fat) tissue, so you may see some symptoms of detox (diarrhea, headache, rash, slight fever) as you release these toxins in the fat you lose.

Once you are at the weight you want to maintain, if you don't want to weigh anymore, use your clothes and how you feel in your own skin to gauge your progress. Use a tape measure to make sure your waist is staying the same. If clothing is getting tight, that is a good way to know you may need to tweak things. The scale is one indicator of health, but it doesn't always tell the whole story. Be aware of all the non-scale victories you are experiencing in addition to progress you are seeing on the scale!

Fasting Schedules

In the 1950's and 60's, and before, people
between the fed state and fasted state. Th
hours out of the day with 3 meals and no
for about 12-14 hours a day. This schedu..
for overall weight management, as long as balanceu
whole foods are being consumed at least most of the time.

If you're trying to lose weight, chances are you will need to
extend your fasting time to see progress. The longer you stay
out of the fed state the longer fat burning occurs. You may start
with fasting 15-16 hours and keep your eating window at 8
hours. Even extending fasts by a few hours can make a
significant difference. Closing your eating window at least 2-3
hours prior to bed is important as well. I open my eating
window sometime between 12-2 pm most days and try to
finish dinner between 6-7 pm. This gives me about 18-20
hours of fasting most days.

After your body adapts to that amount of fasting, you can
extend your fasts to about 22-24 hours, or eating one meal a
day most days. This is helpful to promote weight loss, and just
about everyone will lose weight with this regimen. Which meal
you choose to eat is up to you. Most people who are working
and have families like to choose dinner as their main meal so
they can eat with their families. But, if you prefer to have a
later breakfast or a late lunch and it works in your schedule,
you could eat a big lunch and then fast until the next day's
lunch, or even breakfast to breakfast. The main concept is to be
fasting more hours than being fed so your body is forced to
burn fat stores. I typically eat one meal a day once a week. It
simplifies my life, as I don't need to think about what I am
going to eat all day and frees up a lot of time! You can switch
things up and fast 18 hours 3 days a week and do OMAD (one
meal a day) for 3 days and maybe 1 day a week you eat in the
morning. There is no rule that you have to follow the same
eating schedule every day.

another type of fasting called monthly variation. I
st this for many clients, especially women who are
menopausal or menopausal. As there are 4 weeks in a
month, you intermittent fast for the first week like we talked
about, maybe a fast of 16-20 hours and feast for 4-8 hours
daily. For week 2, you calorie restrict for 1 week. Remember,
you don't want to restrict calories long-term because it doesn't
work. It will gradually lower metabolism if done for weeks and
months. But for one week, it's helpful, so for week 2 you calorie
restrict to about 500-1000 calories per day (500 if you're
smaller, 1000 if you're larger). Week 3 you intermittent fast
like we talked about. Again, you fast for 16-20 hours and feast
for 4-8 hours, or whatever fasting times you are comfortable
with. Finally, the last week of the month you increase
carbohydrate (about 75-100 grams/day) and calorie intake
and that is a feast week. What you are doing over the month is
varying your intake every single week so your body does not
adapt to any one way of eating. It is kept guessing, which
typically stimulates weight loss and overall better health. That
is called monthly variation, and it can be done over and over.

Another example of switching up your eating schedule would
be weekly variation, which is typically what I do. It is called 5-
1-1 or you could do something similar. 5 days out of the week I
fast for about 18-20 hours. 1 day of the week I fast 23-24 hours
and eat one meal a day. The last day of the week I eat in the
morning and have 2-3 meals that day. The reason for this
variation is to force your body to adapt and change.

Change is key!

Try different approaches to intermittent fasting. Give it some
time, at least 1 month. Switch things up if something feels off.
Maybe you are doing the wrong type of fasting or too long of a
fast for where your body is now. This is a healing journey we
are talking about. In three to four months, your body may feel
way differently than it does now, doing the same type of

fasting. Meet your body where it is at, today. Start slowly and follow the guidelines of Nutritional PEACE closely.

Feast days are just as important as fasting days! Sometimes I come across someone who doesn't want to add a feast day in because they are getting results and are afraid of getting derailed. Quite the opposite is true! Feast days remind the body it is not starving, and it will continue to burn fat stores. If your body thinks it is in starvation mode, it will lower metabolism to conserve, regardless or what or how much you eat. *Don't eat less, eat less often!*

Crescendo Fasting

Crescendo fasting is basically fasting for 2, nonconsecutive days out of the week. For example, fasting on Monday and Friday, or Tuesday and Sunday, just not 2 days in a row. On the days that you fast, keep your exercise light, maybe a walk or yoga, nothing too intense. Start with fasting just 12-16 hours, nothing extreme. This will help your body ease into the stress of fasting and reap the benefits if you are more sensitive to fasting.

From there, you can work up to 3 or more days of fasting each week until your body adapts and you feel benefits from fasting. Follow the same guidelines for exercise as you work your way up. Pretty soon you will be fasting 18-20 hours most days without a problem, and feeling great while doing so!

If you're feeling well while implementing crescendo fasting and seeing the results you were hoping for, there is no reason to switch things up unless you hit a plateau. There is no reason for you to be in the top tier of all fasters! This is where your fasting regimen needs to be your own, and you need to listen to your body and be flexible. If you feel great with crescendo fasting and are seeing the results you hoped for, you can stop there. With that being said, it is OK to experiment and change things up as well.

Crescendo fasting works well with those who are very ill and need a fasting schedule that is slow and steady. Those with known thyroid issues also do well with crescendo fasting. Meet your body where it is at and increase as tolerated.

Multiple Day Fasts

This is where people get scared and think, how am I ever going to go multiple days without eating if I am having trouble skipping breakfast?

Don't stop reading! Multiple day fasts can have significant benefits, no matter what health outcome you are striving for.

Multiple day fasts take time to work up to. They work well with those who have a lot of extra body fat to burn off, and also those with diagnosed type 2 diabetes and insulin resistance. I tend to avoid recommending those I am working with to do two-day fasts because day two of a longer fast is typically the hardest. If you can get past day two, fasting gets easier. Hunger starts to fall after day two and you are truly in fat burning mode by the third day. If you extend your fasts to 3, 4 or 5 days, you are getting all the benefits of a 2-day fast, but the days tend to be easier after the second day.

First, glycogen stores are burned and used up by around 24 hours (sooner with heavy exercise), which are stored carbohydrates. Then your body burns limited circulating proteins. It makes the shift to burning fat completely by hours 36-48. If you take in less carbohydrates or your body is used to burning fat, this process is shorter. The longer you are in fat burning mode, the more comfortable your body gets. It's like your body realizes how much fat storage there is and it's like winning the lottery! Your hunger settles after day two, and your metabolic rate goes up, as you are not restricting fuel, you're simply switching from using fuel you are eating to using fuel that is stored. Remember, you still can lose weight and do very well with 16 and 24 hours of daily fasting because the key is really insulin. When insulin falls you will start to burn stored food energy. If you eat a lot of carbohydrates, you will have more glycogen stores and it will take longer to tap into burning fat. As insulin falls, you burn glycogen, but it will also make it easier for your body to access fat stores. If you have had high insulin for a long time that has developed into insulin resistance, it can be more difficult for those with longstanding obesity and type 2 diabetes to lose weight. This is where longer fasts and more intensive strategies are helpful.

Multiple day fasts are not for everyone, but they will help you to meet your weight goals much quicker. Many clients I work with like how they feel during longer fasts and find them to drastically simplify life. You can cycle from shorter fasts to longer fasts, as you are comfortable. If you want to fast longer than 5 days, I would strongly encourage you to work with your doctor for medical supervision.

For each day you fast, you will burn about ½ pound of actual stored fat. So, if you do a 3-day fast each week, you will lose 1.5 pounds of fat every week, or about 6 pounds of fat a month. If you intermittently fast the other days on top of that, you will lose more.

If you choose to do a fast longer than 24 hours, I recommend you put a pinch of sea salt with your water, or drink some pickle juice each day that you fast. Because your body gets rid of sodium and extra water weight as insulin falls, you can avoid cramping and headaches with a little sea salt. For fasts longer than 1-2 days, I recommend an Epsom salt bath each day to replenish magnesium stores as well. Simply add 1-2 cups of Epsom salts to your bath water.

When contemplating longer fasts, you really need to think about what your goals are. Are you primarily trying to lose weight? Reverse diabetes or insulin resistance? Avoid cancer? Increase longevity? Improve gut health? Improve autoimmune illness? If your primary goal is to lose weight or reverse disease of insulin resistance, it makes sense to do longer fasts more often. You could add them in maybe weekly or every other week, or once a month. If you are at a healthy weight and looking to increase longevity or decrease cancer risk, you could extend your fasts maybe seasonally or a couple of times a year. It is really up to you and what you are looking to achieve. If you want to lose weight, do more fasting. What specific regimen you do is up to you.

16, 18, 24 hours, 3-5 days, they all work.

If you ever feel unwell during an extended fast you should eat. You can always try again at a later time. When breaking a long fast, it is a good idea to start with a small meal lower in carbohydrates, maybe a couple of handfuls of nuts, an egg, or a small green salad. Then, about a ½ hour later you can have a balanced larger meal. This will help you to avoid digestive distress and allow your system to slowly working again!

Special Considerations for Women

Several women I have worked with were told by their doctor or practitioner it is unhealthy or unsafe for women to fast. While there are obvious differences between men and women, it makes sense for any body to be in a fasted state. One main difference is that men may have better blood sugar control and insulin sensitivity, so longer fasts can be easier for them.

While this is a controversial subject, it doesn't need to be. Thousands, and even hundreds of years ago, women were forced to fast when food was not readily available, just like men. If you are female and worried about the safety aspects of fasting, it is smart to look at your starting point and particular circumstances. Think about what your goals are and what it is you want to get out of fasting. There is no reason to think fasting is unsafe for women.

If you think about what fasting does for the body, it makes sense why everyone should do it, at least intermittently. Yes, female hormones are in different levels than male hormones, but there are many amazing benefits that women can be cheated out of if they are afraid of fasting or were told not to fast. The healing properties are the same for males and females.

Male or female, it is important to start with shorter fasts and gradually extend your fasting time. Take it hour by hour. Work through one hour, and then try to go another. Some women can easily go without food while others may have a hard time with low blood sugar if they are primarily sugar burners. Remember, being hungry is where the real magic is happening! Very few of us are starving without nutrients. Our bodies will be fine for hours without food; they are nourished.

In looking at the available data, a 20-hour fast with a 4-hour eating window seems to be a great protocol to help heal women the quickest. It ends up being the time span where you are burning through glycogen stores and tapping into fat burning. In other words, your body becomes adaptive at burning fat. The longer this is practiced, the better your body will adapt to burning your stored body fat. You also tap into the initial stages of autophagy, which will be discussed later.

Think of all the free time you will have by implementing daily, 20-hour fasts!

Obviously, this protocol needs to be eased in to, and following my step-by-step program will help you to do that. I know for me my brain was really foggy before I started intermittent fasting. I had a hard time recalling words I wanted to use and felt as if my everyday speech was not as sharp as it once was. As you can imagine, this was very frustrating as someone who regularly works with clients and gives presentations! Fasting clears out the extra glucose floating around so your focus becomes much sharper. Also, your brain starts to use ketones for energy rather than glucose, and it performs very well running on ketones. Once you eat, energy is diverted to the digestive tract for several hours, leaving less energy focus for other places and processes in the body.

When you fast you give your body the opportunity to do what it is designed to do, heal. Who doesn't want that for themselves? Conventional medication mostly masks symptoms, and symptoms are there for a reason. It is your body screaming at you that something is wrong. Don't get me wrong, there is a time and place for conventional medication, but for chronic illness, fasting can heal your body in a way that medications cannot and will not touch.

For women, fasting can help support healing of infertility issues. Infertility can be reversed in many situations. Little aches and pains diminish or go away, memory improves. Skin, hair and nails change and become healthier. There are so many benefits to fasting, that in my mind, it is a huge disservice to tell women they shouldn't do it.

There are some nuances we need to address when it comes to women's hormones and how they relate to fasting. In the years of fertility, women have changes in their female hormones as they move through the 4 weeks of their menstrual cycle.

In the first half of the menstrual cycle (2 weeks), there is a decline in estrogen, which stimulates FSH (follicle stimulating hormone). This is known as the follicular phase. FSH stimulates the follicles in the ovary to grow. The growing follicles stimulate more estrogen secretion. Estrogen then starts to thin the cervical mucus, this tells the brain to pick a follicle to release an egg from.

Halfway through a women's cycle, ovulation occurs. There is a big estrogen surge, which in turn, causes lutenizing hormone (LH) to surge. The LH surge causes an egg to be released. Now the woman is in the luteal phase, which is the second half of the menstrual cycle. The place where the egg is released is called the corpus luteum, and the corpus luteum secretes progesterone.

The first half of a women's cycle is very estrogen dominant, and the second half is very progesterone dominant. This, of course, is what happens in a healthy female with balanced hormones. If any one of these stages or hormones are out of balance, fertility can be compromised and the female may experience a whole host of unwanted symptoms.

If there is no fertilization that occurs, the woman menstruates, estrogen and progesterone both fall, and the cycle starts all over again. The cycle should be very regular during the years of fertility.

All of this comes into play for women, because depending on where you are with your menstrual cycle, there are changes in insulin sensitivity, how fat is utilized, how fat is stored, water retention and muscle building.

In the follicular stage (first half) when estrogen is the dominant hormone, insulin sensitivity is higher. Women in the follicular phase tend to use more body fat during exercise, and more carbohydrate at rest. If you are going to eat more carbohydrate, it is better to do so in the first phase of your menstrual cycle when estrogen is higher. Fat storage is lowered during this stage, and hunger tends to be less with less cravings as there is little change in metabolic rate. There is also less water retention. It is a great time to increase muscle mass as well.

In the luteal stage when progesterone is high, insulin sensitivity decreases. There is a slight increase in metabolic rate, and fat is more utilized as a fuel source. Because metabolic rate goes up by about 100-150 calories, hunger increases as well. Cravings increase. Blood sugars become less stable. It can also be harder to put muscle mass on in the days where water retention is occurring.

If you are female and you feel like you want to eat everything and anything the week leading up to your period, you now know why!

So ladies... every day of your menstrual cycle is a different hormonal profile. Putting the right fuels in on any given day will help your body be its healthiest.

During peri-menopause (about 5 years before menopause), the number of follicles in the ovary drastically diminishes. When there are no more follicles to be stimulated is when menopause occurs. Hormones become very erratic, estrogen will fluctuate all over the place.

In late phase peri-menopause, estrogen and progesterone basically go to levels of 0. There is an increase in visceral fat deposition, and insulin sensitivity decreases and lean mass may decrease. Metabolic rate and thyroid function may decrease. Protein digestion tends to become more difficult as gastric PH rises.

For these reasons, implementing intermittent fasting, especially after menopause, can be very helpful. Also, decreasing carbohydrate intake and increasing fat intake at this point can help with overall body composition.

Keep in mind, estrogen receptors are all over the body, and men make estrogen as well. There are estrogen receptors in the brain, heart, and bones. Estrogen is mainly made in the ovaries in women, but it is also made in fat, liver and neural tissue. The brain loves estrogen, so the cognitive decline women see at menopause is due to the falling estrogen levels they are experiencing.

Estrogen dominance can happen when progesterone levels are too low. This happens when menstrual cycles are abnormal, or women aren't ovulating. Estrogen is typically very dominant in women with PCOS (polycystic ovary syndrome), which will be addressed in a later section of this book. Obese people, those who drink too much alcohol, those with autoimmune disease, or any inflammation could be estrogen dominant

Those who are exposed to a lot of xenoestrogens may be estrogen dominant. Xenoestrogens bind to and stimulate estrogen receptors in the body, causing the body to produce more estrogen. This leads to estrogen dominance.

Xenoestrogens are found in tap water, plastics, phalates, chemicals and pesticides, cleaning products, laundry detergent, perfume, birth control pills, toys, food dyes, nail polish, make-up, non-stick cookware, and personal care products. They can all be endocrine disruptors. In the first section of Nutritional PEACE I have you prepare your body for fasting and decrease obesogens. Using natural self-care products and decreasing endocrine disruptors and obesogens is an important step to healing, and this is why!

You can learn more about xenoestrogens and how they disrupt hormones here:

https://pubmed.ncbi.nlm/nih.gov/12456297/

Anyone with insulin resistance tends to be estrogen dominant.

Men can be estrogen dominant as well, leading to many unwanted symptoms such as increased fat deposition in the breasts (aka, moobs), increased body fat, and overall feminine features. The main behaviors that lead to estrogen dominance in men are too much alcohol consumption, any inflammation, obesity, autoimmune disorders or xenoestrogen exposure.

High estrogen in men typically leads to low testosterone, which leads to erectile dysfunction. A lot of these issues can be fixed with diet and reversing insulin resistance. Men and female hormones can be balanced by following the steps in Nutritional PEACE!

Estrogen (there are 3 types) is a use it and lose it hormone, both in men and women. You don't want it hanging around too long. You want to invite it to the party, have the party and then tell it to go home in your urine or feces! The way you metabolize estrogen is very important. Phase one of estrogen metabolism takes place in the liver, about 70% of our estrogen should be metabolized this way. If you are not metabolizing most of your estrogen in the liver, it is likely a problem of insulin resistance. This leads to the reabsorption of estrogen and estrogen dominance. Again, the underlying issue is likely insulin resistance that needs to be reversed. We can do that!

Women and men alike need to be careful that they are fasting clean as talked about previously. Enjoy the calm of the 20-hour fasted state, but then eat cleanly in your 4-hour eating window. Fasting is not about starvation.

Feasting is just as important as fasting. You can't expect good results if you fast for 20 hours, and then calorie restrict or eat a bunch of packaged processed foods during your eating window. Keep your fasts clean with water, black coffee or herbal tea, then eat whole natural foods that do not come in packages. Fast when you are fasting, and feast when you are feasting. Both are equally important!

What we want to avoid is intermittent fasting creating food phobia in women. I have been there and it is no way to live. Fasting is not about perfection. It is not a diet. It is about connecting with and healing your body. We need to view food as the nourishing and social force that it is. There are always going to be special occasions, birthday parties, vacations, and special events. It is during those times that you need to be ok with being flexible with fasting. You may need to fast 14 hours one day and 20 the next, some days you may not fast at all. Please, please don't sacrifice making a memory with your friends or family because you need to be rigid with your fasts. Have breakfast with your family Christmas morning, eat earlier while on vacation, fast longer when you are ill. Live life!

Women typically have a higher level of the hormone kisspeptin. Higher levels of kisspeptin in women may make them more sensitive to intermittent fasting. If you jump into longer intermittent fasts too soon, it may be too much for your body. Easing yourself in with the 5-Step Nutritional PEACE program will help to combat any issues women may run into.

It works well for women to add in a higher amount of healthy carbohydrates the week prior to their cycle, and if they want to experiment with longer fasts, it is best to implement them the week of their cycle. The higher levels of carbohydrates will stimulate insulin, which can help with thyroid hormone conversions.

If your menstrual cycle is thrown off or goes away entirely, you have hair loss, or you experience less energy, it doesn't mean intermittent fasting is not for you or you should discontinue altogether. You may have been too aggressive with your fasting. An approach you can try if this happens is crescendo fasting, as talked about earlier, or limit fasting to 16-18 hours.

Fasting and Exercise

Please don't misunderstand me, exercise is very important and I have been an avid exerciser since childhood. There are endless benefits to mild and moderate exercise that have been well established, and it is necessary for optimal cardiovascular health. Regular exercise should eventually be part of your lifestyle, if it isn't already.

However, exercise does not play nearly the role in weight gain and weight loss as when and what you are eating. Yes, you read that correctly! Remember, it is the hormones telling the body what to do with the energy you eat that will determine what fuel you are using and what it will be used for.

If you have always exercised in a fed state, it is best to ease into exercising in a fasted state. It is only in the last year that I ever exercised without eating beforehand. I started with low intensity walks of 30-60 minutes and worked my way up to running 3-5 miles while fasting. Then I implemented my regular strength training classes, which last 60 minutes, but are rigorous. At first, I planned to eat shortly after my workouts, but I am a morning exerciser and later trained my body to go without food for several hours after exercising. To my surprise, I felt strong and now prefer running in a fasted state, and not having food in my digestive tract during exercise.

I don't always diet and exercise...

...but when I do, I expect the results to be instant, dramatic & spectacular.

I have run many half marathons, but the last one I completed, I did all my training runs while in a fasted state. My training runs were anywhere from 3-12 miles. I may have felt a bit hungry at the start of some of the workouts, but then the hunger went away and I felt more energetic.

Completing my training runs in a fasted state taught my body how to become fat-adapted, and tap into my fat stores more quickly. When it came race day, I ate breakfast very early in the morning prior to getting to the start line. By that time, I was fat-adapted, plus my body used the extra glucose coming in from eating that morning. Result? A very good half-marathon where I never felt a dip in energy or "hitting the wall"!

Most of the adaptation from using glucose as your primary fuel to using fat for fuel takes place in the matter of a few weeks to a few months. After a few weeks of gentle aerobic exercise in a fasted state, most people can move on to more intense and rigorous workouts such as weight training or interval training. The more you exercise in a fasted state, the better your body adapts to fat burning. It gets better and more efficient over time. When you are able to switch from burning glucose to burning fat, there is really no restriction on how long or how hard you can exercise in a fasted state, because you have hours of energy reserves in the form of fat. You need to be patient over the course of a few weeks to a few months with exercising in a fasted state before your exercise intensity will be the same, or greater than it was in the fed state.

Most people have exercised primarily in the fed state for their entire lifetime! Their bodies are only adapted to using glucose for energy and feel a crash when those stores are used up. Most adults store about 1,500- 2,200 calories in the form of glucose as glycogen. Men have slightly more glycogen than women. If your body is not adapted to burning fat, you will feel a dip in energy when those stores are burned up with exercise. On the other hand, the average human at a healthy weight has 40,000-100,000 calories of stored body fat! Very lean people have less and obese people have much more, which is why extended fasts are helpful. Learning to tap into those stores with intermittent fasting and exercising in a fasted state allows your body to burn stored fat much more quickly and efficiently.

Another important consideration to think about is how quickly you may burn through your reserves of glycogen, and how well you adapt to burning fat when your glycogen (stored glucose) is burned up. For example, if you go for a 60-minute walk in the morning, you may burn about 300 calories. If you have enough carbohydrate stored in the form of glycogen, your body will likely burn that first and after your walk, you will have 300 less calories in the form of glycogen. Your body will then start to utilize stored fat that much sooner.

Remember, there is plenty of stored fat to live off of for several weeks, even in a thin person. Your hormones will dictate which form of energy to use depending on available carbohydrate, protein and fat. Once your glycogen (carbohydrate) is depleted, you may burn a small amount of circulating protein and then, fat! That walk or workout in the morning followed by several hours of fasting will allow the glycogen to be burned up and fat burning to begin. Because you have burned through your glycogen stores and fat is being burned, your appetite will likely be suppressed rather than increased.

You can also split your workouts if you have the luxury of time. Doing cardiovascular training in the morning, fasting all day, then working in some weight training, then feasting on a meal, can be extremely helpful. This will let you burn through your glycogen stores, tap into fat burning, and then use all the nutrients from your meal to rebuild muscles and energy stores. It is very unlikely what you eat will be utilized as body fat storage because the energy you eat will go elsewhere to rebuild. Also, as mentioned earlier, growth hormone will be elevated during the fasting period and muscles will be very receptive to the fuel you put in after your fast.

If you are doing more intensive workouts, say burning more like 800-1000 calories, fasting more than 2-4 hours following your workout can be tough because you have really used up your bank account of energy. In these situations, having a more intensive workout at the tail end of your fasting period, and then eating within an hour or two after your exercise session will likely work better as you are replacing the higher amounts of energy you burned through more quickly.

Timing your workout to end within an hour or two of when you will break your fast seems to be the ideal if your workouts are more intensive and you can work it into your schedule. For example, if you are planning to break your fast at noon, a mid to late morning exercise session that ends around 11-12 would allow the food you eat to directly replenish muscles and energy stores that were burned during exercise. For those following an OMAD pattern, exercising in the late afternoon to early evening will allow for the same thing.

Looking at primal times and how the human body is designed, when blood sugar starts dropping and you don't immediately give your body food, your body responds by priming itself to go and find food. Senses start becoming sharper, your mind becomes clearer, and energy levels actually improve. Your body switches to a different energy system by using fats, also known as ketosis. You use byproducts of fat metabolism for energy rather than glucose, and ketones are incredible fuels for the brain.

Human growth hormone production increases dramatically when you implement intermittent fasting. Intermittent fasting combined with a high intensity training program has shown human growth hormone production to go up by 1,300% in women and 2,000% in men. In terms of putting on muscle, human growth hormone is a very important hormone to increase. Growth hormone allows the body to conserve its muscle during a fast, then rebuild in a feast.

Increased adrenalin from fasting may help you to train harder. At the same time, the elevated growth hormone stimulated by fasting should increase muscle mass and make recovery from a workout easier and faster. This could be an important advantage in elite level athletes, and we are seeing more and more interest in doing this exact sort of protocol, although high-quality studies are lacking.

Growth hormone likely helps in the maintenance of lean mass; both muscle and bone. One of the major concerns about fasting is the loss of lean mass. Some people claim that fasting a single day causes loss of ¼ pound of muscle. Studies prove that this does not occur. In fact, the opposite can happen. In comparing caloric reduction diets to fasting, the short term fasting was 4 times better at preserving lean mass!

https://www.ncbi.nlm.nih.gov/pubmed/1548337

When you give your digestive system a rest, it frees up energy that would otherwise be spent digesting food, and you can utilize that energy for exercise. Digestion requires a huge energy investment by your body. As soon as you eat, your body must stop whatever it is doing and do something with that food. Food is now its main priority. By not overloading the digestive system, your body can use energy for other processes such as detoxification, growth, repair and brain function. Aches and pains and even old injuries can start to heal.

Obviously you need to do what is best for your schedule, and fit in exercise whenever it works for you! We all have families, activities, careers and life to work around. A late morning or late afternoon workout may not work for your lifestyle. Consider your goals, your cardiovascular health and individual schedule. If you are very ill and exercise is not currently manageable, focus on working through the 5 steps of Nutritional PEACE and implement more activity when you are ready.

With all that being said, it works well for some to add in extra carbohydrates the days of heavy exercise to restore glycogen stores. And do remember that protein is easily converted to glycogen as well. If you are used to eating lower amounts of carbohydrates most of the time and add in extra carbohydrates the days of heavier exercise, performance can really improve.

Ultimately, intense exercise in and of itself is very damaging to the body. If you could actually look at your muscles after heavy exercise, you will see they are damaged with micro tears. Massive inflammatory processes take place to clean up the metabolic debris after a rough workout. But then... the body adapts and gets stronger. Exercise, like fasting, is a stressor, but one that ultimately forces us to adapt and change for the better. That is the amazing part of adaptation!

Give yourself 6-8 weeks as an avid exerciser or athlete to adjust to being a fat burner rather than a sugar burner. Make sure your expectations are realistic, don't expect to have perfect workouts and huge changes in body composition the first few weeks you start intermittent fasting.

Diabetes Recovery

Let me be extremely clear. If you have type 2 diabetes and want to reverse this dreadful disease by following the recommendations in this book, you must work with your doctor to do so, especially if you are on insulin or other medications to alter your insulin or blood sugar. It is beyond my scope as a dietitian to help you discontinue insulin safely. Implementing intermittent fasting and reducing carbohydrate intake will quickly decrease the amounts of insulin or medications you need, so it is very important your doctor is onboard with this protocol. *People can and do recover from diabetes* somewhat quickly when fasting is implemented, especially longer fasts.

With that being said, do not be afraid of having this conversation with your doctor! I have known of many patients who have come off insulin and all diabetes medications within a few weeks or months after adapting this lifestyle. Oral medications can be stopped after a discussion with your doctor, but insulin needs medical supervision to discontinue. If your doctor is not open to these suggestions, you can show him/her a copy or this book, or find a doctor or practitioner up to speed and willing to work with you.

There are over 400 million people worldwide with type 2 diabetes; it is a pandemic. It is directly correlated with the changes in our food supply over the past 50-60 years. For the purposes of this book, I will only be referring to type 2 diabetes from here on in, as it is a disease of too much insulin, and a disease of insulin sensitivity. The Nutritional PEACE plan is recommended for those diagnosed with type 2 diabetes, not type 1. Type 1 is an autoimmune disease in which there is little to no insulin secreted due to damage done to the pancreas.

In the American health system, if your fasting blood sugar is 100-125, you are considered prediabetic, and levels above 125 are considered diabetic. For fasting insulin, normal levels are 2-10, and above 10 are considered insulin resistant.

82% of diabetics are overweight and 48% are obese. This is problematic because excessive fat in and of itself is inflammatory. It creates inflammatory cytokines that inflame the entire body. When you fast and lose weight, the inflammation is diminished, which is a huge part of recovering from diabetes.

In type 2 diabetes, the disease of diabetes is a product of years of poor diet, which has led to insulin resistance. High insulin may have even been inherited at birth. Insulin resistance stems from years of pancreatic overload. Over many years, your amazing pancreas has fought a diet high in refined carbohydrates and sugar. It has been overproducing insulin in an attempt to keep blood sugar normal, despite constant incoming bombs of glucose. *When you regularly eat sugar and processed foods, or eat very often, your pancreas is forced to work hard, all the time.*

Your heroic pancreas fights long and hard to constantly keep blood sugar normal, despite a diet rich in sugary foods. Eventually, your body is exposed to too much insulin, and starts to get desensitized to it. As a result, higher and higher levels of insulin are produced to get the same blood glucose control, and energy into your cells.

As I have drilled into your head, when insulin is high, glucagon is kept low. Because your pancreas is fighting so hard to keep blood sugar levels normal by releasing more insulin, an unintended consequence of fat storage becomes apparent, and weight gain becomes very easy. Because excess body fat promotes inflammation, this further contributes to insulin resistance. As the type 2 diabetic gets fatter with poorer blood sugar control, their pancreas has to work even harder to create more insulin to keep up. This results in even more fat storage, weight gain, and further insulin resistance.

Do you see the vicious cycle?

It gets more complicated. In an attempt to control blood sugar, the type 2 diabetics doctor prescribes medications that direct the pancreas to work harder and secrete even more insulin. The poor pancreas works even harder and produces more insulin. Higher insulin means lower glucagon, more weight gain and fat storage, more insulin resistance. At some point the exhausted pancreas can no longer keep up, after trying and trying for decades. When the pancreas fails, the diabetic typically ends up in the ER with symptoms of excessive urination and thirst, blurred vision and headache.

At this point the type 2 diabetic is placed on insulin injections because their defeated pancreas can no longer function on its own. It is too worn out and the body cells are no longer as receptive to insulin. There is now *no limit* to how much insulin a person can inject, and how much fat can be stored, depending on what the doctor has prescribed.

Glucagon does not stand a chance and is kept low and quiet.

It is important to understand that it takes about 10-15 years before you see the effects of diabetes. For example, you could start having higher insulin and glucose in your bloodstream at the tender age of 10, but by the age of 25 when you are diagnosed, a large amount of damage has already been done. Mental confusion, tingling in the hands and feet (neuropathy), brain fog, low energy, long-standing obesity, sexual dysfunction, kidney problems, poor circulation, compromised vision, and accelerated aging are all typically very apparent by the time you are diagnosed with diabetes. If type 2 diabetes is developed and diagnosed in early childhood, it is likely that high insulin levels have been inherited from the mother.

You may be insulin resistant if after more than 4-5 hours without food you experience a lot of discomfort or hypoglycemic-type responses such as headaches, dizziness, intense hunger or cravings, extreme tiredness, or feeling like you need a nap. These are all signs that your body is not responding to insulin and you may be at least mildly resistant to insulin, as glucose is not being taken up by the cells and out of the bloodstream.

Sadly, diabetes is affecting US children at younger and younger ages. If the child has a parent with type 2 diabetes and they live the same type of lifestyle, they have a 70-90% chance of developing diabetes. Yikes, that means almost every child with a diabetic parent will develop diabetes unless changes are made!

Diabetes has a genetic tendency. Think of your genetics as the loaded gun, and your lifestyle, eating habits and environment as the pulling of the trigger. **This gives us hope!** If your family changes their lifestyle and adapts the recommendations laid out in this book, that trigger may never be pulled, even though the gun is loaded.

Fasting is an extremely helpful tool for diabetes recovery. It speeds up a process called apoptosis, which is the body's natural way to destroy dead and dying cells. We want this! The driving force behind diabetes is insulin resistance, but it stems from inflammation. Fasting helps to start healing inflammation almost immediately.

If you are feeling overwhelmed or dejected about the nutritional state we are in today, you are not alone. *However, I am here to tell you type 2 diabetes can be reversed, despite what you likely have been told.* Diabetes is a nutritional disease, and can be corrected with nutritional therapy! Recovering from diabetes means you are off of all medications with a fasting blood sugar of <100. It can be done!

The Nutritional PEACE program is designed to keep insulin and glucagon levels healthy and balanced. Our modern American diet is so perfectly attuned to increasing insulin resistance and obesity it should be criminal to allow such foods to be made and sold! The purpose of this program is to bring you hope, and a natural way to heal your insulin resistance and type 2 diabetes in a very economical way.

I can't wait for you to feel better!

Polycystic Ovary Disease (PCOS)

PCOS is a set of symptoms in females brought on by elevated androgens, which are male hormones. Signs and symptoms of PCOS include irregular or no menstrual periods, heavy periods, excessive body and facial hair, acne, pelvic pain, difficulty getting pregnant, and patches of thick, darker, velvety skin.

Associated conditions include type 2 diabetes, obesity, obstructive sleep apnea, heart disease, mood disorders, and endometrial cancer.

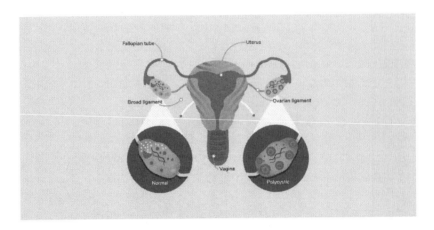

Anovulatory cycles are menstrual cycles where no ovulation occurs. 70% of anovulatory infertility is related to PCOS. During a process called follicular arrest, no dominant follicle grows large enough to ovulate. Without a mature egg, conception cannot occur, leading to the devastating realization of infertility, and that one cannot have a baby.

If you do not ovulate, you can't conceive. Women with PCOS usually have difficulty conceiving, rather than being completely infertile. However, the possibility that you may not be able to conceive a child can lead to severe anxiety. Anovulatory cycles account for approximately 30% of visits to an infertility clinic, of which most are due to PCOS. A heartbreaking 72% of women with PCOS consider themselves infertile, compared to only 15% without PCOS.

The financial costs of infertility are worth noting. Costs range from the relatively inexpensive hormonal treatments (approximately $50 per treatment cycle) to the very expensive in vitro fertilization. The average success rate for one cycle of in vitro, which costs $20,000-30,000 in the US, is only 24.7%. Most women need at least 2 rounds, and not all are successful after the 2nd round. With millions of women suffering from PCOS, the total cost for infertility treatment alone in the United States is $533 million.

Pregnancy loss can be absolutely devastating especially if it was difficult to conceive in the first place. Spontaneous abortions occur in an estimated 1/3 of women with PCOS. Studies suggest that PCOS is associated with up to twice the rate of miscarriage.

Rates of all pregnancy related complications increase in women with PCOS. Gestational diabetes, pregnancy-induced hypertension, and pre-eclampsia risks triple. Risk of pre-term birth is increased by an estimated 75% when compared to normal women or those who have overcome PCOS. Women with PCOS are more likely to deliver by Caesarian section, which itself comes with complications.

In women seeking help with fertility, these treatments may double the risk of multiple pregnancies, and all the complications that accompany more than one baby. Twin births, for example, have up to 10 times the risk of small for gestational age and a 6-fold risk of premature delivery.

During normal menstruation, progesterone is produced after ovulation by the remnant of the dominant follicle. Without ovulation, this does not occur and too little progesterone leads to heavy periods and irregularity. This leads clinically to the irregular cycles found in PCOS.

Interestingly, the underlying cause of the anovulation (no ovulation) relates to excessive insulin and testosterone production. Testosterone is mostly overproduced due to high insulin. I will state that again. **The singular, most responsible culprit for anovulatory cycles is high insulin.**

Weight loss and metformin (a medication given to those with PCOS and type 2 diabetes) improve ovulatory rates, and is the reason metformin is widely used for the treatment of PCOS. All known treatments to reduce insulin, including weight loss, bariatric surgery, and the drugs somatostatin and metformin significantly improve ovulatory function and symptoms of PCOS. Interestingly, patients with type 1 diabetes using high doses of injected insulin also have an increased risk of PCOS.

The three defining features of PCOS include polycystic ovaries, anovulatory cycles, and masculine features. All three symptoms reflect the same pathophysiology — too much testosterone, which is ultimately caused by too much insulin.

Women with PCOS have low levels of the carrier proteins SHBG that bind the testosterone. This amplifies testosterone's effect, even if levels are not particularly high. But what causes this lack of SHBG? T*he culprit is too much insulin.*

Insulin is the major regulator of SHBG production in the liver. The higher the insulin, the lower the SHBG production. This relationship holds true not just in women, but also in men. Decreasing insulin levels through weight loss increases SHBG production.

The striking correlation between blood levels of insulin and testosterone has been noted since 1980. Insulin and testosterone blood levels showed an astounding 85% correlation to each other. High insulin increases testosterone and decreases SHBG, thereby causing the masculinizing features.

If PCOS were just about acne, facial hair growth and missing a few periods, it would not be so devastating! Unfortunately, PCOS is associated with many health concerns, both reproductive and general.

Reproductive issues include:

- Anovulatory cycles

- Infertility
- Disorders of pregnancy
- Fetal concerns

Other significant health concerns include:

- Cardiovascular disease
- Non-alcoholic fatty liver disease (NAFLD)
- Sleep apnea
- Depression and anxiety
- Cancer
- Type 2 diabetes
- Metabolic syndrome

Most women with PCOS suffer from infrequent or absent menstrual periods, mostly caused by anovulatory cycles (ovulation is missed). PCOS accounts for 80% of cases of anovulation leading to infertility.

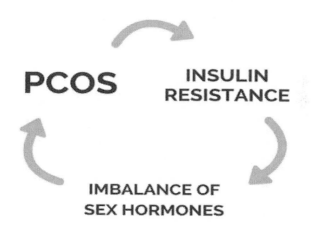

Like obesity, PCOS is best understood as a disease of hyperinsulinemia. This explains the close connection between obesity and PCOS; they are both manifestations of an underlying hyperinsulinemia. They do not always occur together, but are closely associated.

Nutritional culprits, such as excessive sugar and refined carbohydrates, certainly play a big role, but they are not the only factor causing high insulin. The other major factor that increases insulin is insulin resistance. We have learned about this vicious cycle in the section Diabetes Recovery.

PCOS is highly associated with both insulin resistance and hyperinsulinemia. Insulin sensitivity is decreased on average 30–40% in women with PCOS, a degree similar to that seen in type 2 diabetes. Obesity itself is highly linked to insulin resistance, but insulin resistance is also present in normal weight adolescents with PCOS. Independent of obesity, insulin resistance is diagnosed in 75% of lean women with PCOS. In overweight women with PCOS, this proportion increases to an astounding 95%. Essentially, all overweight women with PCOS have evidence of insulin resistance. In addition, normal weight girls with PCOS have evidence of more fatty liver than those without PCOS, another disease associated with insulin resistance.

So, insulin resistance causes high insulin levels, which will contribute to PCOS. But what causes this insulin resistant state in the first place? It turns out to be the high insulin levels itself.

PCOS is really just another manifestation of metabolic disease, caused by too much insulin. This is crucial knowledge, because if the root cause of PCOS (and obesity and type 2 diabetes) is too much insulin, then the solution becomes quite obvious- we lower insulin. We have learned how to do that! The solution is certainly not drilling holes into the ovary. The solution is largely nutritional... decrease processed foods and overall sugary carbohydrates and implement intermittent fasting.

We can achieve this solution by following the steps laid out in Nutritional PEACE!

Additional Health Benefits of Fasting

This section could be an entire book in and of itself, so I am just going to scratch the surface here. Insulin resistance is linked to just about every chronic disease out there- obesity, type 2 diabetes, heart disease, cancer, PCOS, many autoimmune illnesses. This is the result of having chronically elevated insulin levels. Insulin levels are raised by eating too often, and specifically by eating processed carbohydrates and sugars. But insulin will rise no matter what you eat. Carbohydrates stimulate insulin the most, then protein. Fat does stimulate insulin release, but not to the extent that carbohydrates and protein do.

Here is an article titled "Fasting: Molecular Mechanisms and Clinical Applications". Released in 2014, it summarizes some of the benefits of various fasting protocols.

https://www.ncbi.nlm.nih.gov/pubmed/24440038

Inflammation is the common root cause of almost any chronic disease. How can you tell if you are inflamed? You generally don't feel well or have chronic pain. You might experience lethargy, tiredness, and low energy levels. You tend to have weight gain, especially around the midsection. Your body just isn't functioning the way it was designed to. Insulin resistance is seen repeatedly as a common thread to inflammation.

By continuously eating, we always have elevated insulin. Once insulin is constantly elevated, your body is always getting the signal to store energy. Over time, it starts to become unresponsive to the signal to store energy, because the signal is always there. It's kind of like the barking dog next door that really annoyed you when you first moved in, but now the barking is background noise that you have grown accustomed to living with. You learn to ignore it.

Now we have constant insulin circulating all the time. We keep eating 5-6 times per day and drinking coffee with sugar and creamer until late afternoon. Our insulin levels never have time to come down, and glucagon is always quiet. This is where we get insulin resistant, because our body gets desensitized to the constant insulin signal. Over time, insulin resistance leads to obesity, type 2 diabetes, metabolic disease and PCOS as we have learned.

Autophagy

Autophagy, by Wikipedia definition, is the natural, regulated mechanism of the cell that removes unnecessary or dysfunctional components. It allows the orderly degradation and recycling of cellular components.

What?

Thomas Seyfried wrote a book called Cancer as a Metabolic Disease and explains how the body will eat up cancer cells and tumor cells before it touches any good cells. The body is so amazing, it will get rid of dysfunctional cells first. In 2016, a Japanese cell biologist named Yoshinori Ohsumi won the Nobel Prize in Medicine for his research on how cells recycle and renew their content, which is the process of autophagy. Fasting activates autophagy, which helps slow down the aging process and has a positive impact on cell renewal. Here is a link to a summary of his research.

https://www.nobelprize.org/prizes/medicine/2016/press-release/

Basically, autophagy is the process in which old, dysfunctional cells are broken down and those that can still be utilized, are recycled. It is where unneeded protein is broken down and disposed of. When you eat proteins, they are broken down into amino acids, which are basically building blocks. It then uses the amino acids to build more protein and tissue. Anything that is not utilized is converted to glucose, which can then be stored as glycogen or converted into fat.

The practice of fasting used to be criticized because white blood cells start to decrease. Because of this, many thought the immune system could be compromised during fasting. Recent research shows the exact opposite to be true! The body is so intelligent that through fasting and autophagy, white blood cells are destroyed, but they are white blood cells that are no longer functioning optimally. They may be hyperactive or over reactive. The over activity of white blood cells contributing to food sensitivities, allergies or autoimmunity are destroyed. The new white blood cells that are created are less reactive, and can help stop inflammation. This is another reason why fasting helps heal autoimmunity.

If you are well nourished, it is estimated that 50-70% of the protein you eat is actually converted to glucose! Your body does a very good job with recycling the building blocks, so much of what you eat is used for energy instead. If you are very malnourished, you will use all of the available protein to rebuild. In the Western world, much of the protein you eat is turned into glucose.

Autophagy is related to a nutrient sensor called mTOR, which is more specific for protein. If there are lower levels of protein circulating in your body, mTOR will go down, and if you have a lot of available protein, mTOR will rise. When your body senses that it is not taking in enough protein, it will start to break down some of these sub-cellular parts, and utilize them for energy and to rebuild other proteins. Then, when you eat protein, you rebuild and repair what is necessary. See how this is beneficial? You get rid of old, unnecessary tissue while fasting, and then when you eat, you rebuild it new. Instead of taking energy to digest food, now your body has time to recycle, rebuild and repair.

There is now science behind the benefits of fasting, from boosting immunity, to getting rid of dead tissues, and then regenerating stem cells, which is important to maintain health and promote longevity. Your body is very efficient at reusing good materials and getting rid of the bad, if given the chance in a fasted state. This is why fasting is so important to your healing journey and disease prevention. Fasting also lowers insulin growth factors, which are a precursor to cancer.

In adults, growth is not necessarily a good thing. As an adult, your liver shouldn't be growing, lungs shouldn't be growing, and brains shouldn't be growing. Excessive growth is typically problematic. If you're gaining weight, that is excessive growth. Cancer is a disease of excessive growth. Atherosclerosis, which is buildup in the arteries, is also growth. None of it is good!

One way to turn down and disable growth signals is to restrict nutrient sensing pathways. Your body will not excessively grow if there are no nutrients for it. As you fast, if you don't eat any protein or carbohydrate for about 24 hours, your body will start to break down protein. Most people think this is bad, but it is helpful. You are not going to lose muscle just because you are burning protein. Your body is smarter than that. There is a lot of extra protein in the body that needs to go.

If you compare obese people to normal sized people, they have about 20-50% more protein than a lean person. There is excess skin, connective tissue and mass. When you lose weight, you need to burn off all the extra connective tissue, collagen and skin. That is all extra protein. One way to break that all down is through the process of autophagy, which is naturally turned on in periods of fasting. This is why people losing large amounts of weight through fasting do not typically need surgery to remove excess skin... their body has done it for them through the process of autophagy! Some researchers think autophagy may play a role in preventing Alzheimer's disease and cancer, but more research needs to be done to determine how. All of these interesting and amazing effects that you can't simply turn on with weight loss alone can be achieved through autophagy.

As we know, growth hormone rises in periods of fasting. The reason for this is growth hormone is preparing your body to rebuild when you do eat. As you break down protein, your body gets rid of old junky protein that you don't want anyway, unless you are malnourished. Then, when you eat again, growth hormone is high and you can efficiently rebuild protein stores with new amino acids. Nothing turns growth hormone off faster than eating!

In essence, you have done a complete renovation of your body's proteins with long periods of fasting. Think of it this way...Your kitchen cabinets and appliances have been around since the 1970's and you need a remodel. The first thing you do is tear out the ugly cabinets and aged appliances that are breaking your energy bill. You have to get rid of the old stuff that is inefficient before you can place your beautiful new white cabinets and sleek, energy-efficient appliances.

The body is the same way. The first process that needs to happen is breaking down, then you can rebuild the new and better! That is much healthier than keeping the "old junk" around. Autophagy can be thought of as a renewal cycle of protein that only happens once you get to that protein burning stage. Old protein is replaced with new, which can be very powerful. This may be a good reason to consider a longer fast, even if only once or twice a year. I know of people who have completely turned around autoimmune issues and long-standing health issues with longer fasts in moderation.

Many who lose large amounts of weight and body fat worry that they may have problems with loose skin as they trim down. The body gets rid of bad cells during a fast, but it also raises up stem cells to replace the broken down tissue with new tissue. The replacement of the stem cells would tighten the skin and make new collagen and skin cells.

Looking at religions and ancient fasting rituals, there was much wisdom in those practices, which was likely unknown by the people practicing them. The once a year fast to cleanse bodies for religious purposes expended excess glucose leading to diabetes, excess fat causing obesity and excess protein that is now being linked to diseases such as cancer and Alzheimer's.

Fasting is extremely powerful, and best of all, completely free! In fact, you save money, as you are not eating as much or as often. You have more free time to do the things you love! You are preventing chronic disease that you don't even know about. Free disease prevention? No drugs or side effects? Time and money saved? Sign me up!

Cancer Prevention

In the 1920's, Nobel laureate Otto Warburg found cancer cells thrive on the breakdown of glucose. Through a process called anaerobic metabolism, cancer cells burn glucose for energy in the absence of oxygen. Cancer cells prefer this, even when oxygen is available. Cancer is so aggressive that it doesn't wait for oxygen for growth; it will break down glucose without it. Because it doesn't need oxygen, cancer can grow as large as it wants.

Fatty acid metabolism requires oxygen, so cancer cells cannot utilize fatty acids to grow. Scientists theorize the cancer's preference for glucose may be its greatest possible weakness, and a diet low in glucose may help to prevent cancer before it starts.

Being in the state of ketosis and using fat for fuel can be a helpful tool for cancer prevention. As stated, cancer cells can only use sugar for energy, they can't use fat. This allows your immune system to clear out cancer cells while in ketosis, as cancer cells can't make the adaptation to fuel with ketones.

There are some metastatic cancers that can use fat for fuel, but in general, non-metastatic cancer cells cannot make the conversion of using fat instead of glucose. Even the process of bringing glucose really low isn't typically successful in starving cancer down, but fasting can be.

A study in 2016 followed women for about 10 years who had early stage breast cancer. Those who finished dinner earlier and had 13 hours or more of fasting had a 36% lower risk of recurrence of cancer and a 22% lower risk of overall mortality.

https://www.ncbi.nlm.nih.gov/pmc/articles/PMC4982776/

There are currently many randomized studies taking place around ketogenic diets and cancer, including Duke University, Tel Aviv Sourasky Medical Center and St. Joseph's Hospital and Medical Center of Phoenix, AZ. If diets inducing ketosis do in fact protect against cancer, we would expect high levels of glucose metabolism to increase cancer rates. We can utilize ketone metabolism by eating less processed carbohydrates and fasting. The results of these studies may bring exciting nutritional approaches to help the prevention of the awfully devastating disease of cancer!

Brain Function

Fasting is one of the most proven strategies to raise brain derived neurotrophic factor (BDNF). BDNF can activate brain stem cells to produce new healthy brain cells. It enhances brain function, memory and concentration. Fasting may increase BDNF by up to 50-400%.

When you don't eat, metabolism actually increases because your sympathetic nervous system activates growth hormone and adrenaline, which increase brain function. Once you get to a state of burning fat and ketones for fuel you realize, wow my brain is on fire! You don't take so long to remember things, your word retrieval improves, and you don't misplace keys or forget where you park. It's a noticeable difference!

Some experts call Alzheimer's disease type 3 diabetes. It is basically another name for insulin resistance going to your brain, and your brain is not able to utilize fuel efficiently. You get signs of dementia. This eventually leads to inflammation, more free radicals, and more plaquing, which can lead to Alzheimer's disease. Utilizing fats and ketones for fuel is a very clean fuel that generates a lot less free radicals to be utilized by your brain tissue.

Longevity

There are a lot of exciting studies looking at how fasting can increase longevity. If you want to die earlier and age faster, eat all the time and constantly spike your glucose and insulin! The more insulin and glucose spikes you have throughout the day, the earlier you may die.

To increase longevity, don't eat less, eat less often!

A basic principle to increase longevity is to eat a diet with high micronutrient density, which means no excessive calories. Excessive calories, especially empty calories, lay the groundwork for chronic disease and shorten human lives. We want to remove the empty calories, the junk food, the

Frankenfoods, fake oils, fast foods and processed foods. Consistently eating natural foods is critical for keeping us free of chronic disease.

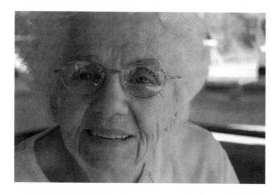

A byproduct of normal metabolism is the creation of free radicals. Normal amounts of free radicals are beneficial as they act as signaling molecules. For example, when you exercise, free radicals are created, which signal physiological benefits such as muscle building. However, an excessive amount of free radicals lead to inflammation and chronic illness, and shorten the lifespan. Eating constantly and eating excessive amounts of processed foods lead to the creation of excessive free radicals.

Another way fasting extends the human lifespan is because it lowers IGF-1 (insulin growthfactor-1), and keeps it low for prolonged periods of time. Lower levels of IGF-1 slow the aging process and increase cellular repair mechanisms. Cells can rid themselves of toxins with lower levels of IGF-1. Excessive intake of animal protein can also elevate levels of IGF-1, which is why it is important to consume plenty of whole plant-based foods. *When we eat all day, we accelerate the aging process and create metabolic inflexibility.*

Autoimmune Illness

Again, I am just going to give a broad overview regarding intermittent fasting and autoimmune disease. There are over 90 types of autoimmune illnesses now identified and named, but not many have known causes (except celiac disease). People are left dealing with their myriad of symptoms for life, and are often times prescribed debilitating medications that cause yet more symptoms.

46 million Americans suffer from autoimmune illness.

I have more experience with autoimmune illness than I would like. Out of the blue, my middle son started having extensive and unrelenting diarrhea in March of 2016. By June of 2016 he was diagnosed with ulcerative colitis, a severe and debilitating form of inflammatory bowel disease. His diagnosis came one day after his 11th birthday. I will not go into great detail how I recovered him here, but I did do extensive research and reading in the area of autoimmunity in the 3+ years that he was severely ill. We tried endless conventional and natural therapies, diets and approaches. He remained very ill for 3 years, becoming steroid dependent and plummeting down the height and weight charts.

Even though there were many approaches that helped minimize symptoms, it was only when we treated my son's ulcerative colitis as an infection with a cocktail of antibiotics that he healed. Within one week he was symptom free with normal lab values. He remains well and symptom free today.

While I am not a proponent of long-term antibiotics, they obviously have their place and saved my sons colon. As a mom, I always had a nagging feeling his case was infection-based. I could barely stomach the immune suppressant infusions he was put on, which were categorized as chemotherapy, and fought to have them discontinued after only a few months. Again, they have their place, but do not address the root cause of why the immune system is overreacting in the first place.

With that being said, it is difficult to pinpoint any one underlying issue for any one autoimmune disease, each case is unique. I do believe there are many underlying issues that could be causing your immune system to react- food proteins, bacteria, viruses, infections, fungi, mold, parasites, heavy metals, toxins, chemicals, or a combination of one or more.

I also believe that fasting is helpful to just about anyone suffering from autoimmune illness. Almost everyone with autoimmune illness can be traced back to having leaky gut, or intestinal permeability. This is where the lining of the gut becomes damaged and large proteins are allowed to leak out into the body where they do not belong. The body sees them as invaders and attacks.

In leaky gut, the GI tract is overwhelmed and overworked. Say you work hard at your job from 9-5. At the end of your shift, you are ready to go home. You get ready to leave and your boss asks if you could just work 4 more hours. So you work 4 more hours, and at the end of that shift you are really wiped and dying to go home. Your boss mandates you to work another 4 hours. By the time you actually get home and go to bed, you sleep a while but are exhausted when you get up, and guess what? You need to go back to work!

This keeps happening. You keep going back to work and your boss keeps mandating you work long hours. You never get a chance to recover and quickly get exhausted and overwhelmed. You can't ask someone to cover for you, because your company is already short-staffed. You are frustrated and ready to quit, but you need the job.

This is what often happens in the case of leaky gut. Your gut is overwhelmed and never has a chance to recover. Either you are eating foods that are unhealthy or inflammatory, or foods you are allergic to. For example, foods high in sugar or processed fats could be causing gut damage. If you eat them all day long you are constantly bombing your gut, and it can only take it for so long before there are problems.

There are also medications that can contribute to gut damage, both over the counter and prescription. Ibuprofen and aspirin can cause intestinal serration and bleeding. My son was instructed not to take any ibuprofen after his diagnosis, as his gut lining was already compromised. Pain medications can cause constipation and block the bowels from properly functioning. Many blood pressure medications can directly damage the gut. Cholesterol medications may lead to an inability for gut cells to restore, repair and heal themselves.

When we look at all the factors that lead to leaky gut, it is no wonder autoimmune disease is on the rise. If we eat too much overall, eat too frequently, eat packaged foods, eat too much in one sitting, are on medications and have out of control stress, we really never give our gut a rest. If we constantly eat processed and packaged foods devoid of nutrition and digestive enzymes, we are asking our guts to digest foods that are very, very hard to digest because the enzymes are not there to help.

The gut is asked to work too long and too hard until it reaches a breaking point. This is where leaky gut happens. Some of the proteins that leak through the gut look like our own tissues, so if a particular protein you are eating (such as gluten) looks like thyroid tissue to your immune system, it may attack your thyroid because it is just trying to get rid of the foreign protein. The immune system basically gets confused and starts attacking its own tissue accidentally. This process is called molecular mimicry and has been well documented since the 1980s.

Your gut needs a break. The fasting mechanism can take away the work the gut needs to do and has been doing, like a much-needed vacation!

This is why eating small frequent meals does not work, for reasons other than it constantly stimulating insulin. Your gut never gets a break when you eat this way! When you get up in the morning and immediately eat breakfast because that is what every health professional has told you, you immediately start assaulting your gut. If it is already compromised, it makes it very hard for you to ever recover. You need to give the gut enough rest for *healing* to occur. This is where intermittent fasting is a very, very powerful tool.

As discussed, women can have a harder time fasting longer periods due to hormonal differences. Males also have more muscle tone, giving them more blood sugar capacity. They can typically pull off longer fasts easier than women. 24, 36 or even 48 hours of fasting can be very healing for men and can relieve a lot of pain.

Women may have a harder time with longer fasts, but 16-20 hours can typically be worked up to without a problem. If you feel your blood sugar is dropping too low, you can actually stimulate your adrenals. If the adrenal glands are already fatigued, you can feel worse. Start with about 16 hours of fasting as discussed earlier, and extend as tolerated. Again, it's important not to restrict calories within your eating window.

Keep in mind that grains, lentils and legumes can be very hard to digest. If you have autoimmune illness or known leaky gut, avoid eating these foods until your digestive tract has healed and you feel well with a lot of energy. I haven't purposely eaten gluten in over 3 years. My grain intake is very limited.

Gluten has been shown to disrupt a protein in your small intestine called zonulin. Your gut cells are like millions of Legos snapped together, and **only one layer thick.** Think of the protein zonulin as the anchors that keep the Legos together. These are called tight junctions. Gluten disrupts the tight junctions and breaks them apart. So, instead of the cells being tightly held together so that nothing leaks through your gut, it can be pulled apart and proteins and other matter coming in from your digestive tract can leak out.

What leaks out goes straight to your immune system, because your immune system is right behind your gut wall. These leaks stimulate and over stimulate the immune system every day. That's part of the precursor in the development of autoimmune disease. It's not that your immune system is ignorant or isn't doing its job, rather, it is over stimulated.

Think of it as a soldier who has been in combat for days and days and is utterly exhausted. After war, the soldier comes back into civilization, but is jumpy and has PTSD. When you have a leaky gut caused by gluten exposure, think of every individual cell and the immune system as being jumpy soldiers with PTSD. It is jumpy because everything is leaking through. It is being constantly activated to defend your body from something it is not supposed to be defending it from. The gut's job is to take the nutrients from food, absorb, and then expel the waste. Nothing within the GI tract is allowed into the bloodstream unless the gut wall says, "yes, you may go through". It is a very intricate process.

However, when the gut is leaky, these checks and balances are broken. The gut's job is to keep anything interpreted as harmful out of the bloodstream and immune system, but it can't do its job when it is leaky. Toxins build up and start to leak into the bloodstream. Remember, when we eat, it is not just food we ingest. There are bacteria's, fungus, viruses and chemicals.

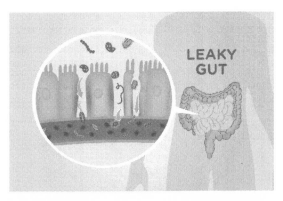

Source: www.biokplus.com

Phalates from plastics, infections, yeast overgrowth, antibiotics, medications, chronic stress, mercury, BPA, pesticides, parasites, and toxic or inflammatory foods can all cause leaky gut. Again, this is why cleaning up your diet and preparing your body for fasting in Step 1 of Nutritional PEACE is so critical.

Although I don't typically recommend using bone broth in the case of weight loss as it can break your fast, it can be helpful for those recovering from autoimmune illness. Making your own bone broth with organic bones will ensure that you are not ingesting chemicals and additives that may make your illness worse. Bone broth can help repair leaky gut, as all the restorative minerals are extracted from the bone marrow of the animal. If you are very ill when beginning Nutritional PEACE, bone broth can be a nice bridge to use with fasting while getting used to longer periods without food.

Most people with autoimmune have leaky gut. Not all, but it is very common to see the two hand in hand. Fasting strategies can be very helpful for people with autoimmune illness that's caused by leaky gut. Lastly, if you are very ill with autoimmune disease, do not exercise too aggressively as it can worsen leaky gut.

Although fasting can be an integral part of healing autoimmune disease, ultimately the trigger that caused the leaky gut in the first place must be dealt with. This is why autoimmune illness can be so complicated, as many triggers may be contributing. For my son, we knew it wasn't directly caused from foods because he followed very strict diets with no inflammatory foods for many months without much improvement. He had no food sensitivities prior to becoming ill, and his illness came on very suddenly. We were not perfect eaters prior to him getting sick, but we certainly ate leaps and bounds above the Standard American Diet (SAD). We also did some heavy metal detoxing. All these things helped, but it wasn't until we nailed his infection with antibiotics that he fully healed from his severe colitis. I am well aware of the implications caused by long-term antibiotics, but in his case, they were necessary.

Even now, we keep him on a gluten free diet with limited sugar or processed foods for the above reasons. Yes, it is hard as a teenager to eat with restrictions, but the food is fresh and eating packaged food is good for no one. I do not allow him to go to many sleepovers to protect his sleep, and we try to keep his stress level as minimal as we can. We have a reverse osmosis system for drinking water, and do not store foods in plastics. Being outside in the sun is encouraged whenever possible.

You can definitely work some fasting into your healing plan, albeit slowly, but if you don't see the improvements you wish, my advice is to find a functional medicine provider who understands autoimmune illness very well and is willing to test you for possible triggers. You can follow the steps in this book for nutritional help, but may need additional testing if your symptoms go beyond healing your gut.

Digestive Issues

This section is not meant to be all-inclusive, but will give you a general idea of fasting and how it relates to gut issues, which can be very complicated. There are studies that have substantiated fasting can help with both IBS, irritable bowel syndrome, and IBD, inflammatory bowel disease, which is sub-categorized into Crohn's or ulcerative colitis, as the main subcategories.

https://www.ncbi.nlm.nih.gov/pubmed/30840892

If you're not eating, you're giving your digestive system a break. Your digestive system does not have to break down and digest. Perhaps you have a lot of food allergens, and eating less often helps you to not expose yourself to the allergens as often. Maybe you had food that was fermenting and putrefying inside your gut, basically rotting inside of you. Now that food is not there if you fast for extended periods. Digestive stress is off your plate, your gut has a chance to relax and heal.

Most digestive issues come in some assortment of gas, bloating, abdominal pain, altered bowel function, either diarrhea, constipation, or an oscillation between the two. In addition, there may be indigestion or reflux. There is generally a myriad of different gut symptoms.

Those who will likely benefit the most from true fasting, meaning no calories in the system as I lay out, are those who have gastrointestinal, neurological, or metabolic imbalances. Symptoms include gas, bloating, loose stools, diarrhea, brain fog, a hard time with memory recall, being overweight, obese, have high blood sugar, high cholesterol, or high triglycerides. Those are a lot of symptoms, but these individuals will likely benefit the most from true fasting, as many of these symptoms stem from imbalances in the gut.

Those who are experiencing symptoms of burnout or high stress load, are not sleeping well, wake up an hour before their alarm clock and they can't fall back to sleep, wake up two, three, four times a night and can't fall back to sleep, are tired during the day, require caffeine, feel wired but tired, or are underweight, this subset of people will probably do best with a *modified liquid fast* that allows them to get some calories into the system. They are likely having adrenal issues, are over stressed or have burnout. In these cases, especially if underweight, you can start with a modified liquid fast for shorter time periods that is very easy to digest and will give the gut a rest. After symptoms begin to subside, you can graduate into longer periods of fasting with no calories. Crescendo fasting would be a next good step.

If you're having gut issues, it is also important to look at what you are putting in that you may be reacting to. Even with fasting, if you continue to put inflammatory foods in that cause your symptoms, they will be less severe, but your gut will have a hard time healing.

I always have my clients start with eliminating gluten, dairy, and sugar completely for **3 weeks** as they are the worst offenders. After 3 weeks, *add 1 back in at a time,* and wait for at least 3 days before after adding another. Note your symptoms when you add a food group back in, as there can be delayed responses. That gluten you ate on Tuesday may be causing your Thursday brain fog. I have followed a gluten free diet very low in grains and sugars for years because I know these foods cause me abdominal bloating and I don't digest them well.

If you still have issues after this, an elimination diet could help, which you can find more information on through the Internet or a registered dietitian.

An elemental diet can be very helpful for those trying to recover from IBD. I wanted to try this with my son when he was very ill, but it was very challenging with his age and going to school. There are two types of elemental diets. There are fully elemental and there are semi-elemental. The semi-elemental diets are likely better for those needing to regain weight. I am not an expert in this area, but here is a good resource and doctor specializing in gut health and recovering from IBD. This is a helpful resource for using liquid and elemental diets.

https://drruscio.com/

When adjusting to fasting or a new diet, a little bit of turbulence in your gut is not abnormal. But the timing of the turbulence or any kind of negative reaction is very important. You may experience a flare of gas, bloating, constipation, abdominal pain, or even things like headache, joint pain, fatigue, or insomnia as a result of something flaring in the gut.

If the adverse reaction lasts for a few days, or up to a week, that is suggestive of some kind of microbial die off or a rebalancing reaction. But if it lasts beyond a week, this may suggest something that you are doing is not working well for your system. If a certain diet or lifestyle implication is not working for you, don't keep going with it month after month, hoping to get over the hump.

As you're going through the healing process, you should expect to feel better when fasting or liquid fasting. You may not feel quite as well when you go back to eating food. But the question is, do you feel the same as you felt before the fast or do you feel like you've made some progress? If you have made some progress, you can continue to fast and heal little by little.

Fasting alone may not be enough to completely rectify gut issues, but it can be extremely helpful. You may never really get to an appreciable level of improvement from just fasting alone. The fasting can be helpful, but you may need to combine it with other therapies, such as metal detox, to reach full healing. Another doctor I would recommend with this process is Dr. Dan Pompa.

https://drpompa.com/

Body Composition

Intermittent fasting can promote huge shifts in body composition, even when changes on the scale are not as obvious. This is why I encourage everyone to take their picture and body measurements prior to starting intermittent fasting, and encourage them to re-measure every couple of months. Seeing changes in inches is very encouraging and an excellent motivator. Avoid weighing yourself too often as sometimes your weight may not change as much as hoped, but you are healing inside during your fasts and losing unwanted body mass. Pictures don't lie!

A 2014 study found that intermittent fasting can lead to weight loss of 3-8% over 3-24 weeks. The same individuals in this study also lost 4-7% of their waist circumference.

https://www.sciencedirect.com/science/article/pii/S1931524 41400200X

When NOT to Fast

We talked about when not to fast regarding hormones. If you have known thyroid or adrenal issues, fasting must be eased in to. If you are under a high amount of stress, your first focus should be reducing stress and balancing nutrition. Staying in step 1 of Nutritional PEACE is critical for your success until you feel well enough and have enough blood sugar stability to work in regular intermittent fasting. As you get healthier with proper nutrition, fasting can become an option for you. Crescendo fasting can be a good place to start.

Once you have enough blood sugar stability to make it 16 hours or so in a fasted state and feel well while doing it, you can begin to intermittent fast regularly. Start by fasting on days that are not as stressful or active for you. Fast sporadically on days you feel well and have less stress, don't feel as if you need to fast every single day. Start with fasting 1-2 days a week and make sure you are eating enough calories within your eating window.

Don't fast if you are pregnant or nursing. This does not need a lot of explanation. Your hormones are all over and you are growing another human! Eat regular meals daily until you are completely finished with nursing, and even then, give yourself a few extra months for hormones to level out before you begin intermittent fasting. With that being said, if you feel nauseous or skip a meal here or there while pregnant, it's not the end of the world and your body will feed your baby necessary nutrients.

If you have an active eating disorder or have struggled with years of disordered eating, make sure you are in a place where you are applying intermittent fasting for health improvement, not because you need to be obsessive about what you eat. There is a fine line between being disciplined and being way too stringent. It is important you fully recover from disordered eating prior to starting any fasting strategy.

Children, in general, should not fast as they are still growing. There are ways to help them lose or stabilize their weight if they are struggling with obesity or insulin resistance. You can apply a lot of the same principles that are outlined above, but make sure they are eating 2-3 meals daily with balanced nutrition. Take out most sugar and starchy foods that are not nourishing. Eliminate snacks in between meals, especially packaged and processed foods. Provide water as their main beverage and keep sugary drinks and juice very minimal. Unless they are practicing or playing a sport later into the evening, there is no need to eat after dinner.

Obviously, children can have some treats and enjoy special occasions. But keep the special occasions special, not daily!

There are always exceptions. One of my success stories, Paige, implemented a lot of the guidelines for intermittent fasting at age 16 to clear her acne. She took her breakfast to school and ate it in class around 10, rather than before she left for school. She avoided eating after dinner, and significantly decreased her intake of processed carbohydrates and sugar. Water was her only drink the vast majority of the time. On special occasions with her friends, she was sure to enjoy treats she normally didn't eat, because that is part of being a teenager. Within 3 months, her acne completely healed!

PART 3- WHAT TO EAT

What to eat has been at the forefront of nutrition education as the main focus of weight management for several decades. As we have learned, the timing of and how often we eat is as important or possibly more important than what we are eating when it comes to balancing our insulin levels. This single change will likely stimulate weight loss for just about everyone, along with a myriad of additional health benefits.

However, what we eat is obviously important too! Our food system has changed so dramatically over the last 40-50 years that our bodies have not been able to adjust. Processed and fake foods are at the core problem of insulin resistant disease. Highly processed food is also highly palatable, so here poses an enormous problem between knowing what is nourishing and craving what isn't. Processed foods provide little satiation and are very difficult to stop eating. Because there is so little nutrition, your body keeps craving and wanting real food and nutrients that don't come.

The SAD (Standard American Diet) is 55% calories from processed foods and 33% from animal products. That doesn't leave us with many whole, natural plant foods! The American diet is made up of predominantly low nutrient, processed foods that are high glycemic (cause a high insulin spike).

Real food provides a variety of natural colors, different nutrients, and fiber. It also TASTES GREAT and provides fullness. Cravings diminish because you are actually feeding your body what it needs, which is real food full of nutrients.

Time-restricted eating helps with reducing and eliminating cravings. Because you are more focused on eating within a restricted time frame, having to decide what is "good" and what is "bad" isn't as important. If you crave sweets after meals, have some sort or sweet food or dessert, just do it within your eating window. You are still having that sweet something, but it is timed within your window at the tail end of a meal. Rather than eating your meal and then having a dessert 2-3 hours later before bed, you are still enjoying your sweets, but you are implementing 2-3 hours of fasting time that helps to keep your insulin levels balanced.

The reason we start with preparing your body in Nutritional PEACE is because that will bring you the most success. What you do outside of fasting is just as important as the fast itself. If you are binging on junk food and processed fake food while feasting, you will be ravenous and hungry, even hangry, during your fasting window. This is because you are never giving your body the nutrients it needs. We start with preparing your body by taking out all the junk, because this will start to calm your inflammation, heal your gut, and increase detoxification pathways. Then we implement the next natural step of intermittent fasting.

Please hear me, you cannot intermittent fast your way out of a processed foods diet! You just can't. If you don't eat nutrient dense foods during your feasting window, you will struggle during your fasts.

One life simplifier that I love is not having to think about or clean up breakfast. Bypassing breakfast shreds about 20-30 minutes off of my busy morning routine. It also means bypassing all the junky breakfast foods such as pastries, cereal, toast, French toast, waffles, bagels, donuts, sugar-laden yogurt, muffins, juice, and breakfast cookies. It is all highly processed "food" that gives you an enormous insulin spike with very little nutrition. Once you understand how insulin and glucagon work, you know how defeating it is to eat a load of sugar every morning.

My most important lesson that took me way too long to learn after practicing in the field of nutrition for 20 years, is that no diet works, and every diet works! There just isn't a perfect diet for everyone because we are all metabolically individualized with a unique genetic makeup. Our environments, stress levels, sleep habits, family life and overall health have a profound effect on how we will absorb and utilize nutrition. You could eat the cleanest diet, but if you have a chronic disease or leaky gut, you won't utilize the nutrition in the same way as if you were in better health.

One easy way to think about improving your overall nutrition is to take the food guide pyramid that has been entrenched in our brains for decades and invert it! Instead of having 6-11 servings of bread, pasta, cereals and grains, keep these minimal. There is no nutrient in processed, starchy grains that cannot be acquired from whole foods. Instead, have an abundance of colorful vegetables and ample healthy fats. Focus on fats such as coconut oil, avocados, olives, olive oil, nuts and seeds. A favorite nut of mine is macadamia, because it is lower in protein and very satiating. Keep protein moderate, because that stimulates insulin as well, and excess protein is converted to glucose (glycogen).

With that being said, here are some general recommendations that will help you to heal your body and take advantage of both your feasting and fasting times.

Nutritional Variation

Diet variation is very, very important. It is too easy to get into a food rut and eat the same thing every day. I was guilty of this myself! I remember eating either oatmeal or a whole-wheat bagel with peanut butter and a banana most days for breakfast for years. I did this even though I felt horribly bloated by early afternoon, almost every day. I bought the same things over and over at the grocery store, because I thought they were healthy and it was predictable.

Let's talk about seasonal, monthly, and weekly variation. This will help you to rotate the foods you are eating, and ensure your body is getting a variety of nutrients. These variations will also help to bring the body not only different nutrients, but also break up the monotony of eating at the same time and doing the same routine every day. When the body is given different foods, food groups and daily routines, it is forced to adapt and become stronger.

The easiest way to create nutritional variation is to eat what is in season. Avoid eating produce that has been sent halfway around the world and picked well before it ripens. Depending on where you live, this might keep you a bit more limited during certain seasons. Where I live in Wisconsin, we have a surplus of lettuces, fresh garden vegetables, berries, cherries and melons to choose from in the summer. Fall is harvest time and we can focus more on squash, apples, grapes, and root vegetables such as potatoes, beets, and carrots. Winter brings citrus fruits. While they are not grown in Wisconsin, at least they are coming from a shorter distance and are picked when they are ripe. Spring is great for asparagus, strawberries and mushrooms.

When you eat seasonally, you ensure that you rotate nutrients found in a variety of foods that are available. Find a local farm market and buy as much produce there as you can.

When you eat seasonal foods, you also tend to take in a different proportion of macronutrients. Because there are so many more fruits available in the summer, we tend to take in a higher amount of carbohydrates. This tends to be OK because most people are more active in the summer months. In the winter, humans traditionally ate more smoked foods and fats that were stored, as fresh produce was not available.

Varying the diet helps to ensure you feed your gut microbiome well. Your microbiome is made up of trillions of bacteria in your large intestine. We know that this bacterium comprises at least 70% of your immune system. When you feed your microbiome a variety of fresh, seasonal foods, the bacterial balance can flourish.

Your microbiome can change in a matter of days, depending on what you feed it. Studies show eating high amounts of sugar and highly processed foods for even a few days feeds harmful bacteria, allowing it to overgrow and crowd out healthier bacteria. This means eating the Standard American Diet can compromise both your immune system and overall health. Eating enough fiber and whole foods feeds the bacteria that is considered helpful in keeping your microbiome in balance.

It is never too late to change the health of your microbiome for the better! When the microbiome is constantly fed different foods, it is forced to change and adapt, and that is where the magic is.

Monthly Variation

We have talked about monthly variation already, but I do want to touch on one different type for those who may have thyroid issues, as they don't always do well on lower carbohydrates or jumping into intermittent fasting too quickly. However, they do seem to benefit from short bursts of higher carbohydrate. For females, eating higher carbohydrates the week of their menstrual cycle is a good way to cycle in short bursts of healthy carbohydrates. Men could pick one week a month to implement the same strategy. It is important to focus on nutritionally dense high carbohydrate foods such as whole fruits and berries, sweet potatoes, sprouted grains, wild rice, squash, and root vegetables. Avoid processed carbohydrates with little nutrition.

By increasing healthy carbohydrates one week a month for those with hormonal challenges can help you make hormone conversions. The elevation of carbohydrates while intermittent fasting for a short period increases insulin, putting you in a more anabolic (building) state. After that week, intermittent fasting with lower carbohydrates can help stimulate weight loss and overall healing again.

Weekly Variation

Although we know chronically elevated insulin increases inflammation and ages you prematurely, we also need to pay attention to insulin levels that are too low for too long. We could look at someone who has been on a very low carb diet, such as keto, for a very long time. They initially got results, but then all of the sudden start gaining fat around their waist and losing muscle. Their diet has not changed in months.

What is happening?

Very low insulin levels for a long time can actually shut off gluconeogenesis (converting protein to glucose). We don't want that to happen! When insulin goes really low for a long time, there isn't enough insulin to shut off gluconeogenesis, and you can actually lose muscle.

How do we counteract that? With monthly (
That's it. Elevate the insulin short-term so
is not starving. Pick 1-2 days a week or 1
higher amounts of healthy carbohydrat
intermittent fasting. It's a fine line. If you e.
elevate insulin all the time, you will store fat. Bu.
of carbohydrates are magical, as the body will then b.

If you have a lot of gut issues and find yourself intolerant to carbohydrates, you can eat high protein instead as weekly or monthly variations. Protein elevates insulin almost as much as carbohydrates, and will work with the variation as well. Pick 1 feast day a week and eat 2-3 meals that day. Once you are well on your way to an intermittent fasting lifestyle, it may be hard for you to eat 2-3 meals per day, but doing it only weekly, or a couple of days a month is important.

A **weekly variation schedule** would look something like this: 5 days per week eat 2 meals per day, maybe in an eating window of about 1-6pm. Then one day a week eat OMAD, or go from dinner to dinner without eating. Then feast on Saturday or Sunday!

This is an example of a weekly variation schedule I recommended to a client who was *brand new to intermittent fasting:*

Week 1:

Fast 13-15 hours 5-7 days, 1-2 days feel free to eat breakfast, choosing a day when you are more active, avoiding snacking in between meals and at least 3 hours before bed

Week 2:

4-5 days practice 15-16 hours of fasting, pick 1-2 days to fast 16-18 hours

3:

days practice 18-20 hours of fasting, 1-2 days 16-18 hours, day feel free to eat breakfast, choosing a day when you are more active

Week 4:

Try 1-2 days OMAD (one meal a day), 6-7 days 18-20 hours of fasting

Pick 1 day each week to cycle in higher amounts of healthy carbohydrates, about 75-100 grams that day (sweet potatoes, peas, carrots, potatoes, beets, sprouted grain bread, rice, dried beans), OR incorporate more carbohydrates the week prior to your monthly cycle

~ You can be flexible with this schedule, implement what works in your lifestyle! Cycle through again every 4 weeks.

This is an example of **weekly variation** recommendations I gave to a client who was *much further along in the fasting process* and was used to implementing regular, 3-day extended fasts. She initially had a large amount of weight to lose. She needed some variation in both her nutrition and intermittent fasting schedule.

To vary your intermittent fasting schedule, try something similar to this:

Week 1:

3 days OMAD (one meal a day), 3 days 18-20 hours of fasting, 1 day feel free to eat breakfast, choosing a day when you are more active

Week 2:

2-3 days OMAD, 4-5 days 18-20 hours of fasting

Week 3:

3-day fast, 3 days 18-20 hours of fasting, 1 day feel free to eat breakfast, choosing a day when you are more active

Week 4:

1-2 days OMAD, 6-7 days 18-20 hours of fasting

~ Pick 1 day each week to cycle in higher amounts of healthy carbohydrates, about 75-100 grams daily (sweet potatoes, peas, carrots, potatoes, beets, sprouted grain bread, rice, dried beans)

This type of schedule keeps the body guessing, as fasting is not predictable. Also, the cycling in of higher carbohydrates every once in a while helps the body to remember how to use glucose for energy and also may help with thyroid hormone conversions.

Partial Fasts

Partial fasts can be another powerful tool, as they are another form of variation. Remember, when your body is forced to adapt to different things to maintain homeostasis, the unpredictability can promote weight loss and improve overall health.

Pick 5-7 days in a row out of the month where you only eat 500-1000 calories daily. Those of smaller builds can stay closer to 500 calories, and those of larger builds, 1,000 calories. Yes, this is a form of calorie restriction, but it is short-term so your metabolic rate will be protected. Then, for the next 3 weeks eat 2-3 nutrient-dense meals daily without snacking. Repeat this monthly. Again, your body is kept guessing, which will promote weight loss, but preserve metabolic rate. This is another good way to transition in to longer fasting periods.

Now we will discuss more in depth which actual foods and food groups to focus on during your feasting times.

Keep Sugars and Processed Carbohydrates Minimal

Now that we know that nutritional variation is extremely important, let's look at the actual types of foods we can focus on to keep our nutrition balanced and optimal. The most important thing you can do when it comes to your diet is remove processed foods. By this time you are likely tired of me repeating this, but processed foods really are sabotaging. Sugar, white flour, bagels, croissants, pancakes, crackers, soda, donuts and similar foods are very dangerous. Refined carbohydrates are easy to become addicted to because there are no natural satiety hormones released after we eat them to tell us we are full. Refined foods are not natural foods, they are highly processed. *Their toxicity lies in the processing.*

Sugar stimulates insulin secretion, but it is much more detrimental than that. It also promotes fat accumulation by increasing insulin both immediately and over the long term. Research shows that sucrose and high fructose corn syrup promote fat storage more than any other foods. Sugar is uniquely "fattening" because it directly produces insulin resistance. With no nutritional qualities, added sugars should be the first foods eliminated (or nearly eliminated) in any eating plan. The addition of sugar to processed foods provides almost magical flavor-enhancing properties at virtually no cost.

This is why packaged foods can be so dangerous, and hard to give up once you are hooked on them.

Naturally occurring and added sugars are distinct from each other. The two key differences between them are amount and concentration. Sugars are often added to foods during processing or cooking, and sugars may be added in unlimited amounts. Also, sugar is often present in much higher concentrations in processed foods than in natural foods. Some processed foods are virtually 100% sugar. Fruits with natural sugars contain fiber, and dairy contains protein and fat to help make you feel full. Fruit and dairy also provide us with many other nutrients. Processed foods with added sugar often contain no dietary fiber to help offset any harmful effects. For these reasons, efforts should focus on reducing **added** rather than natural sugars.

Keep in mind, sugar is not always labeled as sugar. Other names include sucrose, maltose, glucose, fructose, dextrose, molasses, hydrolyzed starch, honey, cane sugar, invert sugar, high fructose corn syrup, brown sugar, corn sweetener, rice/corn/can/maple/malt syrup and agave nectar. These aliases attempt to conceal the presence of large amounts of added sugar.

A popular trick by the food industry is to use several different names and types of sugar on the food's label. This trick prevents "sugar" from being listed as the first ingredient and leads us to believe the product isn't primarily sugar.

We are smarter than that!

Focus on Fiber

Insulin and insulin resistance drive obesity, this we now know. Refined carbohydrates such as white sugar and white flour spike insulin the most. With this being said, carbohydrates are not inherently fattening, they only become toxic after they are processed.

Today, many diets label carbohydrates as villainous. Carbohydrates that God made for you in their natural form will affect blood glucose and insulin levels very minimally. Fiber is the missing part of processed foods, stripped by food companies, causing our once harmless carbohydrates to become empty and harmful calories.

Fiber is essential in sending fullness messages to your brain. It also helps move food along your digestive tract quickly, essentially "cleaning" the large bowel. Just more reasons to eat whole, intact fruits and vegetables in their natural forms!

Our body's fuel with nutrients from natural, unprocessed foods. By taking fiber and other components out of foods, the balance is completely destroyed. For thousands of years humans ate carbohydrates in their natural form, with little to no obesity, diabetes, cancer, or disease.

Many plant foods have changed over the past several decades. We do not eat the same species of wheat as our descendants of long ago. Today, an estimated 99% of all wheat grown worldwide is dwarf or semi-dwarf variety, as it brings higher yields. The dwarf wheat varieties are not the same as those of fifty years ago. There has been a change in nutritional content due to soil management and pesticide use. An obvious clue to the changes in wheat is the skyrocketing of celiac disease and other digestive issues of gluten intolerance.

Wheat flour is ground into such a fine dust that its absorption in the intestine is extremely rapid. This amplifies the insulin effect. Whole-wheat flours are absorbed almost as quickly. Wheat is converted to glucose more efficiently than almost any other starch.

The main problem associated with processed wheat and carbohydrates is the decrease in fiber intake. Fiber is not digestible and is only found in plant foods. It is either in a soluble or insoluble form. Soluble is found in berries, oats, dried beans and avocado. Insoluble can be found in leafy vegetables, whole wheat and whole grains, flax and nuts. Fiber gives food bulk, and soluble fiber absorbs water to form a gel, which gives it even more volume. Chia seeds are a prime example of this, anyone who has ever had one caught in their teeth knows how it quickly absorbs liquid and forms a gel!

Fiber also increases stool bulk, as it is not digestible, and helps with excretion in the colon. Unfortunately, fiber intake has decreased significantly over the centuries. Humans were estimated to eat 77-120 grams of fiber each day in Paleolithic times! Traditional diets of a century ago were around 50 grams of fiber. Sadly, modern American diets only contain about 12-15 grams of fiber daily.

Virtually all plant foods in their natural, unrefined states contain fiber. Fiber has the ability to reduce absorption and digestion, which is good for insulin control. Western diets have one defining feature- the amount of processing of foods. Fiber is removed to increase shelf life. It is removed from frozen foods because it expands when frozen, which poses a problem with food manufacturers.

Natural plant foods have a balance of nutrients and fiber that humans have evolved to consume. Removing everything except the simple carbohydrate destroys the delicate balance of the plant, and makes it toxic for us to consume. Nor are our bodies designed to handle foods with chemical additives.

Ultimately, consuming plenty of whole plant foods will ensure you take in the proper amounts of fiber for optimal health, but you must focus on eating them in their natural, unprocessed forms.

Facts About Fructose

Fructose is the main sugar found in fruit and is considered the sweetest naturally occurring carbohydrate. Before the 1960s, natural fruit consumption contributed small amounts of fructose to our diets, about 15-20 grams daily. By the year 2000 it contributed to 9% of total calories in the Standard American Diet, with adolescents taking in an average of 72.8 grams per day!

High-fructose corn syrup was developed in the 1960's as a liquid sweetener. It was cheaper to process than sucrose, which was processed from sugar cane and sugar beets. High-fructose corn syrup could be processed from the masses of cheap corn grown in the American Midwest. As a liquid sweetener, it was extremely easy to mix into processed foods. In addition, it is sweeter than glucose, prevents freezer burn, helps browning, and extends shelf life.

As a result, high-fructose corn syrup has made its way into almost every processed food. Big Food companies use it because it is cheap and plentiful. Interestingly, fructose has a low glycemic index, meaning it doesn't cause a big spike in blood sugar. It only mildly raises insulin levels compared to glucose. However, almost every cell in the body can use glucose for energy, but NO cell has the ability to use fructose.

Once inside the body, only the liver can deal with and metabolize fructose. Glucose can be utilized for energy all over the body, but fructose is shunted directly to the liver. Excessive fructose puts enormous pressure on the liver, as other organs cannot help metabolize it. Excess fructose is converted to fat in the liver, and high levels of fructose lead to a fatty liver for this reason. Fatty liver leads to the development of insulin resistance in the liver. Fructose over consumption often leads directly to insulin resistance, which leads to type 2 diabetes and obesity.

If the liver is already full of fat because fructose keeps coming in at high levels, insulin tries to force more fat and sugar into the liver because it has to go somewhere. The liver is already full of fat and sugar from overeating processed foods and eating too often. It gets more and more difficult for insulin to shove more glucose and fat into a fatty liver. It then takes more and more insulin to move the same amount of food into a fatty liver. The body then becomes resistant to the efforts of insulin since normal levels of insulin are not enough to push sugar into the liver.

A vicious cycle ensues. If insulin levels start to drop when you don't eat, stored fat and sugar comes rushing out of the liver and the body keeps raising insulin levels to deal with the energy coming out of the liver. Your liver wants to get rid of the extra energy, but the energy causes insulin release.

Obvious sources of fructose are high fructose corn syrup and fruit. Agave nectar, once touted as a healthy and natural go-to sweetener should be avoided, as it is higher in fructose than sugar. Honey is almost identical to table sugar chemically. It is a mix of glucose and fructose, which will quickly stimulate your blood sugar and insulin levels. Honey does contain a bit of fiber and some healing qualities, but raises insulin too quickly to heal insulin resistance.

Because fruit is wrapped in fiber and other nutrients, it does not pose the same threat as soda or processed foods. However, in someone recovering from obesity and insulin resistance, I recommend keeping fruit minimal, about 1-2 servings daily, and only fruit in its natural form.

This is why it is so important to remove added sugar and processed foods from your diet, and step 1 of Nutritional PEACE is to prepare your body for fasting.

Eat A Healthy Fat Source at Every Meal

Of the 3 macronutrients (carbohydrates, fats and proteins), fat is the least likely to stimulate insulin. So... fat is not inherently fattening, but potentially protective! Strive for a higher proportion of natural fats. Natural, unprocessed fats include olive oil, butter, coconut oil, beef tallow, olives, avocados and avocado oil, organic whole dairy, and lard. Nuts and nut butters are also high in fat, with significant health benefits. They are naturally high in fiber and low in carbohydrates.

Full-fat organic dairy is delicious and can be enjoyed if tolerated. Studies show that full-fat dairy is actually associated with a 62% lower risk of type 2 diabetes. Avocados have been recently recognized as a very healthy and delicious addition to any diet. High in vitamins and potassium, avocados are very low in carbohydrates and high in monounsaturated fat. They are also high in both soluble and insoluble fiber. These fibers keep your colon happy!

Our available fats have changed dramatically over the last century. Almost overnight, millennia of eating beef tallow, pig lard and churned animal butter began to be replaced by a non-food seed oil, highly chemically altered to be heat stable. In 1940 it was discovered how to create seed oils such as soybean, canola, safflower and sunflower, which were stable enough to sit for long periods on grocery shelves. Later, these oils were rebranded as vegetable oils to obscure their true source, seeds.

Following the work of a researcher by the name of Ancel Keys, the American Heart Association began to recommend saturated animal fats be replaced with processed vegetable oils in 1961 and 1971. Butter and lard was replaced with margarine and trans fats (trans fats have now been banned from our food supply because they are so toxic!). Saturated fats have been demonized ever since.

Sadly, there was no data to support the transition to the use of highly processed seed oils, and there remains no data today. On the contrary, there have been hundreds of well-organized, randomized controlled studies, which have shown that replacing saturated fats with vegetable oils does not improve cardiovascular mortality. In actuality, there have been numerous studies, which have linked diets high in processed oils with higher incidences of inflammation, cancer, gallstones, stroke and cirrhosis of the liver.

There is no need to avoid and be suspicious of the foods God made for you. Instead, be leery of refined and processed carbohydrates full of sugar and processed fats, and foods made in a factory. These foods have contributed far more to the problem of heart disease than all of the entirety of saturated fats throughout human history.

Vegetable oils are extracted under intense heat. They turn a very ugly greyish color and have an obnoxious odor. Because of this, they have to be chemically treated to deodorize their smell and then chemically treated again for clarity, and dyed a false golden color.

Today, about 76% of processed American foods contain vegetable oil and nearly 100% of fast food restaurants use them. Vegetable oil consumption has increased 1,400% since 1960!

In the normal human diet, poly-unsaturated fats are found in almost all plant matter as well as in animal meat. They become toxic in their industrial conversion to plastic bottles of mass-produced oil, bought in bulk by grocery stores and Big Food, and cooked into processed foods full of sugar and food parts. God created these oils in foods naturally for us to consume, but humans pulled them out and processed them in a way that made them harmful.

One last thing to note about fats is the ratio of Omega 3 fatty acids to Omega 6 fatty acids. Omega 3's are found in fatty fish and marine life. Omega 3's are thought to help with brain function and staving off dementia. Omega 6's are found in seeds and grains, and extremely plentiful in the American diet. They are prevalent in wheat, corn, soybeans and barley.

When too high, Omega 6's in unnatural forms have been linked to whole-body inflammation. While Omega 3's reduce inflammation, Omega 6's promote it. If in balance, Omega 3 and Omega 6 have a healthy ratio. In the preindustrial era, the Omega 6 to Omega 3 ratio was around 2:1. In 1960 it had climbed to 3:1. After the worldwide spread of vegetable oils and processed foods, it is now estimated that the ratio of Omega 6 to Omega 3 in the American diet is 76:1! This ratio screams inflammation.

Many people supplement with Omega 3's, thinking they can bring their ratio closer. If you are eating the Standard American Diet (SAD) you will never overcome the 76:1 ratio with supplements. You need to drastically reduce your intake of unnatural Omega 6's by avoiding processed vegetable oils and processed foods.

Instead, focus on healthy fats in their natural state that I have already recommended: coconut oil and coconut products, grass fed butter, beef tallow, olive oil, avocado oil and avocado, organic whole dairy products, organic eggs, nuts and natural nut butters and organic meat.

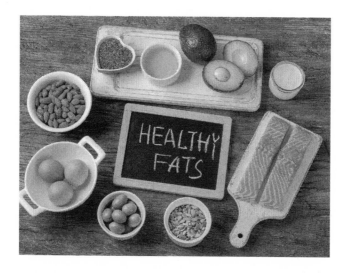

Eat Moderate Sources of Healthy Protein

Protein cannot and should not be eliminated from your diet, but it is important to remember that protein stimulates insulin almost to the same degree as carbohydrate. That being said, protein is the building block for most major processes in your body. Eat a protein source every time you eat a meal. Meat, eggs, dairy, nuts, nut butters, and dried beans are all good protein sources. Protein should make up about a third of what you are eating. Protein is recycled in your body every day, so you do not need to be excessive about your intake either! If your skin, hair and nails are healthy, chances are you are taking in enough protein.

Proteins are highly variable in their capacity to stimulate insulin. For the purposes of this book, it is important to ultimately consume protein in its natural form as much as possible. If able, consume meat and dairy that is grown organically and close to home. An egg produced by a chicken that free ranges is a much healthier choice than a protein bar that has been highly processed with 5 different kinds of added sugar.

chart will help to ensure you are feeding your body
er nutrients each time you sit down to a meal. In addition,
make sure you are drinking plenty of water each day to stay
hydrated, about half your weight in ounces. If you are
overweight, drink about half of your ideal body weight in
ounces. This chart is **not** all-inclusive, it is more meant to give
you an idea of how to balance your meals to meet nutritional
needs.

Fat (1-3/meal)	Vegetable (1-3/meal)	Fruit (1-2/day)	Protein (1-3/day)
Butter (grass fed)	Leafy greens or lettuce	Berries, any	Eggs
Coconut oil or coconut parts	Peppers	Melon	Organic Meat
Avocado	Tomatoes	Pears	Nuts/Nut Butter
Olive Oil	Carrots	Apple	Organic
Avocado Oil	Beets	Orange	Whole Dairy
Whole Dairy or Cheese (organic)	Celery	Banana	Fish/Tuna
Eggs	Cabbage	Grapes	Dried Beans
Nuts/Nut Butter	Cauliflower	Kiwi	Cottage Cheese (whole milk)
Olives	Broccoli	Mango	
Sour Cream (no additives)	Onions	Pomegranate	
	Mushrooms	Cherries	
	Brussels Sprouts	Grapefruit	
	Asparagus	Passion Fruit	
	Cucumbers	Guava	
	Eggplant	Pineapple	

Starches in their natural state such as sweet potatoes, potatoes,
dried beans, organic rice, peas, turnips, rutabagas, and quinoa
can be enjoyed as long as you tolerate them. Some people have
more trouble breaking these down. Try to keep your servings
of these foods to about 1-2 per day, as tolerated. Dried fruit
should be eaten in limited amounts, as the natural sugar
content will be much higher per serving.

General Guidelines/Medication Use

In general, especially to stimulate weight loss, focus on eating a healthy fat every time you sit down to a meal. Take in moderate amounts of protein and lower carbohydrate foods that are rich in fiber. This way you will not over stimulate insulin, but will still be taking in necessary nutrients.

Many people worry about excessive protein being taxing on the kidneys. This is true only if you are not eating enough alkalizing vegetables. Eating too much animal protein can cause your body to become more acidic, and the answer to balancing this out is to eat a lot of vegetables, especially leafy vegetables. Vegetables naturally alkalize the body.

Your body is more responsive to insulin later in the day. One of the worst things you can do for weight loss is get up and eat large amounts of carbohydrates, and that is what most people do! Even eating a large bowl of fruit with yogurt or a big bowl of oatmeal in the morning hours is hard on the body, especially if you are not hungry. The body is more responsive to insulin later in the day, so having more carbohydrates later in your eating window will allow your body to utilize these nutrients better.

Unless you are doing an extended fast, it is important to eat until complete fullness at least one meal out of the day. If you are following OMAD, make sure you eat enough and eat nutrient dense foods for your one meal. If you eat 2 meals, you can make one smaller and in a shorter time frame, but then eat your other meal to fullness. If you calorie restrict during your eating window, you may eventually slow your metabolism, as your body will think it is starving. That is the last thing we want!

Keep in mind fats create less stimulation of insulin. Proteins stimulate insulin a little bit more, and carbohydrates (mainly processed) stimulate insulin the most. Cutting out starchy and processed carbohydrates is critical in reducing overall insulin, as well as not eating as often. The next step is to focus on moderate protein. This is why ketogenic diets work well for weight loss; you're cutting out the biggest stimulators of insulin. Fats tend to be somewhat neutral when it comes to stimulating insulin, but they still will to a certain degree.

If you are having trouble with hunger and cravings when implementing intermittent fasting, adding 1-2 TBSP of butter or coconut oil to your coffee or tea in the morning hours can be a good bridge for a few weeks to help your body adapt to longer periods of fasting. This will give your body a small amount of nourishment with little insulin stimulation.

Be careful to break your fast gently, especially if you have been on an extended fast. Overeating right after fasting can give your digestive system a real jolt, causing stomach discomfort and indigestion. Try breaking your fast with a handful of nuts and a small salad to start. Then you can eat a larger meal within 30-60 minutes.

Remember to ride out your hunger; it will not persist as it comes in waves. Staying busy during a fast day is helpful. As you become more accustomed to fasting, you will burn stores of fat and your hunger will diminish. On longer fasts, hunger often diminishes or goes away completely after day 2.

Be sure to stay plenty hydrated during your fast to avoid any feelings of dizziness. You should not become forgetful or have lower energy, in fact, most report more mental sharpness and higher levels of energy while fasting. If you have any muscle cramping, remember to soak in an Epsom salt bath. If you are experiencing any headaches, add in extra salt to your water.

You may experience less overall bowel movements, or not as much mass when you do go. This is OK! You are eating less often and your body is utilizing what does go in much more efficiently. If you experience any constipation, make sure you are drinking plenty of water and eating fiber and plant foods in your eating window.

If you are taking any medications, be sure to discuss with your physician before starting this protocol or discontinuing taking them. Some medications, such as aspirin or iron supplements may cause problems on an empty stomach. Metformin, used for diabetes and PCOS may cause nausea or diarrhea. If medications absolutely have to be taken with food, you can try taking them with a serving of leafy greens.

Blood pressure may change while fasting, so you may become light-headed if you take blood pressure medication. Consult with your physician about adjusting your medications until you can safely come off of them entirely.

Remember, if you are diabetic and taking diabetic medications, especially insulin, *you must be followed closely by your doctor.* Fasting obviously reduces blood sugars, and if it becomes too low it can be life threatening. Close monitoring of your blood sugars is mandatory. You can expect your blood sugars to come down after implementing this program, so if you have repeated low blood sugar readings, your medication needs to be lowered and the program is working! Blood sugar responses are unpredictable, so close monitoring by a physician is essential.

Persistent nausea, vomiting, dizziness, fatigue, high or low blood sugars or extreme tiredness are not normal with intermittent or extended fasting. Hunger and constipation are normal and can be managed.

Alcohol

The general recommendation I give regarding alcohol is to stay away from it as much as possible when trying to lose weight and improve health. It is inflammatory to the stomach and digestive tract in just about any shape or amount. Within the body, ethanol is converted to acetyl-CoA, which can generate glucose, amino acids or fat. It is the combination of insulin with this precursor to fat from ethanol metabolism that leads to extra fat around the middle (the infamous beer belly). Ethanol combined with carbohydrate can quickly lead to fat storage and weight gain.

We obviously don't make the best choices when alcohol is in the mix, so it can be very detrimental to those trying to lose weight or maintain a fasting schedule. An entire week of intermittent fasting and balanced eating can quickly be sabotaged with binge or late night drinking, especially if it leads to poor food choices.

With that being said, I know not everyone will adhere to this advice, so I will tell you the best way to incorporate a small to moderate amount of alcohol into your lifestyle. Try to enjoy your alcohol within your eating window, and preferably toward the end of your eating window with a meal. Stick to lower carbohydrate drinks such as dry wine or a mixer made with plain seltzer water. Sweet wine, beer and mixers with regular soda are very high in carbohydrates and will stimulate insulin much quicker and in greater amounts. Sorry, beer drinking friends!

Artificial Sweeteners

Artificial sweeteners have long been an area of conflicting data and are heavily studied. Do artificial sweeteners cause an increase in insulin? It depends...

Studies have shown sucralose to raise insulin levels by as much as 20%, despite the fact that it contains no calories or sugar. This has been shown for other artificial sweeteners, including stevia. They may even raise insulin higher than table sugar in some people! Artificial sweeteners decrease calories and sugar, but not insulin, and we know insulin is the main driver of obesity, insulin resistance and diabetes. Since artificial sweeteners raise insulin in many people, there really is no benefit to using them.

Artificial sweeteners have also been shown to increase cravings. Because your brain perceives sweetness, but there are no calories, you may overcompensate with increased appetite and cravings. Furthermore, most controlled trials show there is no reduction in calorie intake in people who use artificially sweetened foods and beverages.

Artificial sweeteners are not found in nature so they should always remain suspect. One of the harmful effects that has been shown is the disruption of bacterial balance in the gastrointestinal tract, and to a pretty large extent. Disrupting bacterial balance may lead to whole-body inflammation, mental disturbances and obesity.

A large multi-study review completed in 2016 compared the effects of the major artificial sweeteners (aspartame, sucralose, saccharin, and stevia) on insulin, blood glucose, and weight gain. The review showed differing and often contradictory results between all completed studies. Again, it depends on the person and how they metabolize the sweetener. Because of all the variables and chemicals, I encourage you to avoid artificial sweeteners whenever possible.

Here is a link to an abstract of a study that looked at sweet tastes and insulin release. Insulin release is referred to as CPIR for "cephalic phase of insulin release".

https://www.ncbi.nlm.nih.gov/m/pubmed/17510492/

One last concept to note is that artificial sweeteners that are found in packages and bags often need to be bulked up with maltodextrin, which is a form of sugar. Because artificial sweeteners are so intensely sweet, the little packets are 96% sugar and only 4% artificial sweetener. Powdered bags used for baking are the same. The primary ingredient is maltodextrin to add bulk to the bag, and ensure baking instructions similar to sugar.

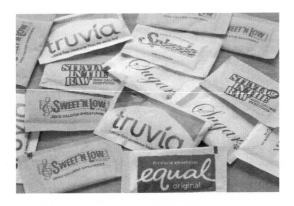

If you do choose to use an artificial sweetener, it is better to use the liquid forms of Splenda or Stevia, which do not contain added sugar.

Many products are sweetened with sugar alcohols, which are chemically modified sugars. They are not as sweet as regular sugars, so are used in much higher amounts. Because they are not digestible in the GI tract, cramping, gas and diarrhea can result. I myself suffer abdominal bloating after ingesting sugar alcohols, so I stay far away from products that contain them. The most common sugar alcohols are sorbitol, mannitol, maltitol, erythritol, xylitol and isomalt.

All of these sugar alcohols have been shown to increase blood glucose, which will in turn, stimulate insulin. For this reason, I recommend you avoid them.

PART 4: NUTRITIONAL PEACE

We made it to my favorite part of the book! Here is my 5-Step Nutritional PEACE program laid out for you step-by-step. Set aside 12 weeks to complete the program. It's OK if you have deadlines, events or vacations during this process. My program is meant to work seamlessly with your lifestyle, no matter what life is throwing at you. In the pilot program that I did, we started in October and ended the end of December. We worked through Halloween, Thanksgiving and Christmas with success! Participants were thankful they had control over their eating during the holidays for the first time in decades.

Some books or gurus will say it's OK to eat anything you want during the time your eating window is open. While there is some truth to this, having the mindset that you can eat anything you want any day of the week, as long as you are in your eating window, can be rather dangerous. I am not saying you cannot enjoy a piece of birthday cake or eat earlier than you usually would for a special occasion, or splurge on lunch at your favorite Italian restaurant once a year. The problem is, some people turn "special occasions" into daily occurrences. "It's OK for me to drink 3 glasses of wine most days because I work so hard. I can eat an extra piece of pizza and drink an extra beer because I ran 2 extra miles. I fasted all day so I am going to reward myself with 2 cookies after dinner."

Again, I don't want you to be so strict that eating is not enjoyable, or you can't be flexible enough to experience life to its fullest. I do want you to be careful in your mindset and view treats as treats and special occasions as actual special occasions. As we have learned, eating food void of nutrients will make it hard to sustain any sort of regular fasts.

I am so excited for you to get started, because I know this program works if implemented as outlined, one step at a time!

If you follow the steps, you will ease your body into this lifestyle little by little, making it effortless to maintain. Do the steps in the order I have them for the duration I allow for your best chance at success! It has taken me 20 years and thousands of clients to figure this out, but I am confident this process will work for you, and you will be feeling better in a few short weeks.

P- PREPARE Your Body

Weeks 1-2

Before diving deep into balanced nutrition and intermittent fasting, we need to do some preparation. Think of it as cleaning the fish bowl prior to putting new fish in. Spending a few weeks clearing out the junk will help your body to adapt to intermittent fasting much easier. Fasting does not work well if you are not eating healthfully. You will be defeating the purpose of fasting if your body doesn't have the right nutrients to heal. Fasting cannot accomplish its miraculous self-healing abilities until it has the right nutrients within the body to work with and build on.

If you are currently eating a lot of processed foods, or eating very often, this phase is necessary and important for long-term success! You need to start flooding your body with nutrients to make sure your body is well nourished before you think about fasting. If you are used to burning sugar as your primary fuel, you need time to transition away from utilizing a lot of refined carbohydrates. Getting rid of the refined foods first makes fasting a lot easier, and helps you to transition to fat burning.

Eating toxic food after a fast can defeat the benefit of the fast, because now you are rebuilding with unhealthy food. After a fast, you absorb and assimilate a greater proportion of what you are eating, so it is critical to replenish with high quality food to build back cleaner and healthier tissue.

If you don't take the time to come off of the Standard American Diet and jump right into fasting, you may feel ill and experience headaches, shakiness or itchiness. These are all withdrawal symptoms, as the liver needs time to detoxify. A lot of toxins can be stored in fat tissue because your body sees that as the safest place to put them. Taking a few weeks to really clean out the junk in your diet is important.

There are four concepts to focus on during the two weeks spent preparing your body:

1. Look for foods that are Non-GMO and Organic whenever possible
2. Avoid Obesogens and Endocrine Disruptors
3. Stop eating at least 3 hours before bed
4. Quit snacking and drinking anything but water in between meals

These 4 steps will lay the groundwork for you to start extending your fasting times in Step 2.

Concept 1:

Purchase and Eat Non-GMO and Organic Foods

GMO stands for genetically modified organism. GMOs are essentially living organisms whose genetic material has been artificially manipulated in a laboratory through genetic engineering, creating combinations of plant, animal, bacteria, and virus genes that do not occur in nature or through traditional crossbreeding methods. Most GMOs have been engineered to withstand the direct application of herbicide and/or to produce an insecticide.

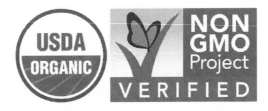

The use of toxic herbicides like Roundup (glyphosate) has increased 15 times since GMOs were introduced. While the World Health Organization announced that glyphosate is "probably carcinogenic to humans," there is still some controversy over the level of health risks posed by the use of pesticides. GMOs are also commonly found in U.S. crops such as soybeans, alfalfa, squash, zucchini, papaya, and canola, and are present in many breakfast cereals and much of the processed food that we eat. If the ingredients on a package include corn syrup or soy lecithin, chances are it contains GMOs.

While Roundup has been banned in many countries and some US cities, the vast majority of crops and plants are sprayed with it. Sadly, Roundup contaminates almost all drinking water, and its by products are found in virtually all human blood samples that are tested.

While the U.S. Food and Drug Administration (FDA) and the biotech companies that engineer GMOs insist they are safe, many food safety advocates point out that no long term studies have ever been conducted to confirm the safety of GMO use. Some animal studies have indicated that consuming GMOs may cause internal organ damage, slowed brain growth, and thickening of the digestive tract. GMOs have been linked to an increase in food allergens and gastrointestinal problems in humans.

For these reasons, it is best to stay away from GMO's until the research is clear!

Eat Organic When Possible!

The term "organic" refers to the way agricultural products are grown and processed. While the regulations vary from country to country, in the U.S., organic crops must be grown without the use of synthetic pesticides, bioengineered genes (GMOs), petroleum-based fertilizers, and sewage sludge-based fertilizers.

Organic livestock raised for meat, eggs, and dairy products must have access to the outdoors and be given organic feed. They may not be given antibiotics, growth hormones, or any animal by-products.

How your food is grown or raised can have a major impact on your mental and emotional health as well as the environment. Organic foods often have more beneficial nutrients, such as antioxidants, than their conventionally grown counterparts and people with allergies to foods, chemicals, or preservatives often find their symptoms lessen or go away when they eat only organic foods.

Grass fed butter compared to conventional butter has 6x the amount of linoleic acid and 10x the amount of Vitamin A retinol, just to name one example!

Organic food is often more expensive than conventionally grown food. But if you set some priorities, it may be possible to purchase organic food and stay within your food budget. Also, when intermittent fasting is implemented, you won't be eating as often, so you can allow your budget to include organic items as you will be saving money overall.

Think about it as an investment, invest in your health now and avoid spending money on sickness care later!

Organic produce contains fewer pesticides. Chemicals such as fungicides, herbicides, and insecticides are widely used in conventional agriculture and residues remain on (and in) the food we eat.

Organic food is often fresher because it doesn't contain preservatives that make it last longer. Organic produce is often (but not always, so watch where it is from) produced on smaller farms near where it is sold.

Organic farming is better for the environment. Organic farming practices reduce pollution, conserve water, reduce soil erosion, increase soil fertility, and use less energy. Farming without pesticides is also better for nearby birds and animals as well as people who live close to farms.

Organically raised animals are NOT given antibiotics, growth hormones, or fed animal byproducts. Feeding livestock animal byproducts increases the risk of mad cow disease (BSE) and the use of antibiotics can create antibiotic-resistant strains of bacteria. Organically raised animals are given more space to move around and access to the outdoors, which help to keep them healthy.

Organic food is GMO-free. As stated, Genetically Modified Organisms (GMOs) or genetically engineered (GE) foods are plants whose DNA has been altered in ways that cannot occur in nature or in traditional crossbreeding, most commonly in order to be resistant to pesticides or produce an insecticide.

As mentioned above, one of the primary benefits of eating organic is lower levels of pesticides. However, despite popular belief, organic farms do use pesticides. The difference is that they only use naturally derived pesticides, rather than the synthetic pesticides used on conventional commercial farms. Natural pesticides are believed to be less toxic, however, some have been found to have health risks. That said, your exposure to harmful pesticides will be lower when eating organic.

Where the organic label matters most:

According to the Environmental Working Group, a nonprofit organization that analyzes the results of government pesticide testing in the U.S., the following fruits and vegetables have the highest pesticide levels so are best to buy organic:

Apples, Sweet Bell Peppers, Cucumbers, Celery, Potatoes, Grapes, Kale, Summer Squash, Nectarines, Peaches, Spinach, Strawberries, Cherry Tomatoes, Hot Peppers

Fruits and vegetables you **DON'T** need to buy organic if on a budget:

Known as the **"Clean 15",** these conventionally grown fruits and vegetables are generally low in pesticides. In many cases, the outside rind or core is not eaten, where there are more pesticides.

Asparagus, avocado, mushrooms, sweet potatoes, cabbage, sweet corn, grapefruit, cantaloupe, eggplant, kiwi, mango, onions, papaya, pineapple, sweet peas

Remember, if the product you select is labeled organic, it is automatically non-GMO. If it is not organic, at least look for the non-GMO verified symbol that is included on products that are GMO free.

Organic meat is important to purchase whenever possible. Toxins, chemicals and anything injected into animals bio accumulates in muscle and animal tissue. When we eat meat and animal products that are conventional and not organic, we are exposed to much higher amounts of toxins that were ingested by the animal we ate. Also, conventionally fed animals often eat genetically modified grains that are rancid and filled with environmental toxins. Eating animals that have been fed an organic diet and are pasture-raised will have much less amounts of toxins when eaten.

Concept 2: Avoid Obesogens and Endocrine Disruptors

According to Wikipedia, obesogens are foreign chemical compounds that disrupt normal development and balance of lipid metabolism, which in some cases, can lead to obesity. Obesogens may be functionally defined as chemicals that inappropriately alter lipid homeostasis and fat storage, change metabolic set points, disrupt energy balance or modify the regulation of appetite and satiety to promote fat accumulation and obesity.

In other words, obesogens are chemical compounds that are added to foods and products that disrupt the natural function of your body and lead to greater fat storage or obesity.

Yikes!

As you can see, it is important to avoid these, and most people have never even heard of this word, let alone know what foods or products obesogens are contained in. Some endocrine (hormone) disruptors have been shown to be obesogens, or involved in weight gain, and may be contributing to the obesity problem in this country. The term obesogens was coined around 2006, based on the knowledge that exposures during early development to specific chemicals were fou[...] normal metabolic processes and increase suscep[...] weight gain across the lifespan.

Obesogens do not directly cause obesity, but they may incre[...] the sensitivity, or susceptibility, to gaining weight, especially when the exposures occur during development. They also disrupt the endocrine system as they bind to hormone sites, making them unavailable for your natural hormones.

Obesogens are believed to work in several ways. They may change how a person's fat cells develop, meaning they may increase fat storage capacity or the number of fat cells.

Also, obesogens may make it more difficult to maintain a healthy weight, by changing how the body regulates feelings of hunger and fullness, or increasing the effects of high fat and high sugar diets.

Some general advice:

- Eat fresh fruit and vegetables; choose organic when possible to reduce pesticide exposure
- Reduce use of plastics, store food in glass
- Do not use plastics in the microwave
- Purchase furniture that has not been treated with flame retardants
- Choose fragrance-free products or natural fragrance
- Avoid foods and beverages that have been stored in plastic containers
- Use stainless steel or quality aluminum water bottles rather than plastic
- Do not feed your babies from plastic bottles, use glass bottles instead
- Instead of non-stick cookware, use cast iron or stainless steel
- Use organic, natural cosmetics and self-care products

Concept 3- Stop Eating at Least 3 Hours Before Bed

This is pretty self-explanatory! There is really no reason to eat after dinner, unless you have medication that needs to be taken with food. In that case, talk with your doctor and explain your situation and ask if you could take it at a different time.

This includes not drinking beer, alcohol, or anything with calories that could stimulate an insulin response.

This is the first step toward narrowing your eating window and have success with intermittent fasting!

Concept 4- STOP Snacking!

We have learned this concept already, but it warrants repeating. Stop eating between meals! The only thing you should be putting in your mouth in between meals is water, black coffee or plain tea. Many foods and drinks that we are told are healthy- kombucha, a handful of nuts, energy bars, MCT oil, kale chips, should not be consumed in between meals or out of your eating window if at all possible. Yes, these foods are nutrient-dense and have their place at meal times, but not in between.

Remember, every time you eat anything with calories, insulin is released and your cells are told to store energy. Eat until you are FULL at meal times, and you should be fine for at least 4 hours in between. This allows your insulin to begin to fall again. Sipping on kombucha or freshly squeezed juice will create a constant insulin release, so limit yourself to water in between meals.

The "healthy snack" is one of the greatest weight-loss deceptions. The myth that "grazing is healthy" has attained legendary status. If we were meant to "graze", we would be cows! Grazing is the direct opposite of virtually all food traditions.

Snacks are often little more than thinly disguised desserts. Most contain high amounts of refined flour and sugar. As you know, these pre-packaged conveniences have taken over grocery store shelves everywhere! Are snacks necessary? No. Keep them out of sight. Ask yourself, am I hungry or bored? There is a simple answer to the question of what to eat at snack time... Nothing! Don't eat snacks, period.

Simplify your life.

Wait until you are truly hungry to eat! Sometimes I fast until late afternoon and then eat a big meal. I am not typically hungry at dinnertime if I do this, and guess what? That is OK! You don't have to let the clock dictate when you eat. If you aren't hungry, it's fine to skip a meal, or eat just a little. That is what your body is programmed to do! I promise you will be fine if you go without dinner. Kids used to be sent to bed without supper all the time as a punishment, although I would not recommend this. They lived!

E- EXTEND Fasts

Weeks 3-4

This is where things start to come together and you will see obvious changes, whether it is weight loss or other non-scale victories (NSV). You have taken the toxic and processed foods out of your diet and replaced them with nutrient dense foods to flood your system with healing nutrients. You are drinking water, black coffee or herbal, unsweetened tea.

By now, because you are not eating after dinner and not snacking, you are ready to start extending your fasts. It took me a couple of months to get used to fasting 18-20 hours most days. It took me several weeks to get used to working out and running in a fasted state. I started slow and worked my way up. I started with walking for exercise in a fasted state, and worked my way up to running and increasing my mileage. I now attend strength training classes in a fasted state. I gave myself time to work up to these activities. If I felt weak or unusually hungry after a run or strength class, I ate. There is no rule that says you have to keep fasting if you are feeling weak, dizzy or unwell. Tomorrow is a new day and you can try again!

Start with at least a 12-hour fast, which you should be doing by now. After that, start pushing back the time that you break your fast in the morning. Push your fast back to 14 hours for a few days, then to 15 hours, then 16 hours and so on.

18-20 hours of fasting works well for many people. You start to see the benefits of autophagy, you have likely burned up glycogen stores (especially if you have exercised) and you are starting to burn fat. Extending your fasts to 22-24 hours will bring more fat burning.

I wouldn't start extended fasts just yet. Remember, fasting is a stressor on your body, albeit a healthy one, but still a stressor. You want to give it some time to adjust.

Get comfortable with fasting somewhere between 16-24 hours. After several weeks, you may start extending your fasts if all is going well. If you have had obesity and insulin resistance for many years or decades, extended fasts can be very helpful. Do not be afraid, your body knows what to do. You may always work with me individually if you need help and guidance during an extended fast.

A- ALTER Nutrition

Weeks 5-8

This is the time I want you to take a hard look at your nutrition. Go back and read the section about what to eat and make sure you are feeding your body nourishing foods at each meal. Go through these questions one by one and answer them truthfully. If you aren't where you want to be nutritionally, use the next 4 weeks to tweak your nutrition and really focus on consuming wholesome foods during your eating window.

I encourage you to take 1-2 hours a week and plan out what it is you will be eating from day to day. You should have fewer meals to plan with intermittent fasting- bonus! Many people want me to write meal plans for them, but I avoided putting general meal plans in this book, because everyone has different nutritional needs, tolerances and preferences. I cannot put a one meal plan fits all out for everyone, it just doesn't work. Remember, all diets work and no diets work! It depends where you are starting at nutritionally, your overall health and what your particular body needs. Some people do very well on a vegan diet, at least for a while, some feel great on paleo or keto. I myself followed a vegan diet for about 6 weeks and felt terrible, because I don't tolerate grains or a lot of carbohydrates very well. However, my best friend might feel great following vegan, or maybe keto.

What I don't want you to do is categorize yourself into any one "camp" and feel as if you need to follow that one style of eating forever, and expect everyone else to eat the same way as you do. Once we do that, we typically miss out on nutrients and may lack complete food groups. We get ourselves into trouble by thinking we have to completely eliminate certain foods forever, unless you have an allergy or intolerance.

What I do want you to do is eliminate packaged and processed foods as much as possible. Avoid sugar and processed fats.

They really have no place in our food system. Believe me, I understand how difficult it is to stay away from these foods, but do try to keep them minimal. Eating seasonally and locally as discussed above should be one of your highest nutrition goals. Rotate the foods and food groups you are eating, find a local farmer for meat who treats his livestock well and feeds them an organic diet. This link will help you find farmers in your area so you know exactly where your meat is coming from! Just type in where you live, and bam! A list of local organic farmers will come up.

https://www.localharvest.org

Think about where you were before starting Nutritional PEACE and where you are now... ask yourself these questions and adjust your nutrition needs and goals accordingly.

Is your eating plan working for you?
Are you still eating processed foods?
Is there variety in your diet?
Are you getting enough fat?
Do you include a fat or fats at each meal?
Are you trying new foods?
Are you eating seasonally?
Do you have a high amount of energy?
Do you feel well?
Do you have a plan for when you eat out?
Are you sleeping soundly?
Do you have any digestive issues?

While it is not necessary to eat nutrient dense foods 100% of the time, the more often you do, the better you will feel and the easier your fasts will be. There are many books and eating plans that say you can eat whatever you want within your fasting window. While this is true to a point, it is not ideal and you will never be in optimal health if you continue to eat foods devoid of nutrients on a regular basis. Save treat foods as "treats", not daily foods! After a while, you won't crave these foods anyway, because intermittent fasting will help restore appetite control. Your body will crave nutrient dense foods instead, especially because you are eating less often and need to make it count! Progress... not perfection!

C- CLEAN, CHALLENGE and CHANGE

Weeks 9-12

Clean:

We are going to focus on three concepts over the next four weeks. First we will make sure during our fast we are fasting clean with no chemicals or additives getting in the way of our success. Take a look at what you are consuming or drinking during your fasting period.

While some practitioners or resources may say it is OK to consume artificial sweeteners, flavored waters that are calorie free, or herbal tea with a sweet flavor, I say leave them for your eating window. Multiple studies on all sorts of artificial sweeteners and their relationship with insulin are conflicting. While Person A may not have any sort of insulin response to diet soda, Person B may secrete insulin because of the sweetened flavor. Even though there are no calories metabolized by the body, the sweet sensation in the mouth may be enough to stimulate insulin and break your fast. Everyone is different. All artificial sweeteners have been tested for insulin response, and they are all over the board depending on the person.

I know of people who drink diet soda during their fast without a problem, and I know of people who add stevia to their coffee and struggle to maintain weight loss. I say why chance it? Fasting clean is important and will help you to maintain mental toughness and clarity.

Some people will add butter, MCT oil or coconut oil to coffee to make it "Bulletproof". While this can be a good bridge when you are just starting out if you are struggling with severe hunger during your fast, you are likely stimulating insulin at least a little bit. You can try this method for a few weeks, but then try to wean yourself off and then make your fasts clean.

YES	NO	MAYBE
Plain Water	Artificial Sweeteners	(I Would
Black Coffee	Flavored Coffee or	Avoid!)
Black or Green Tea,	Tea	Fruity or Sweet
Unflavored	Diet Soda	Flavored Tea
Sparkling Water,	Stevia	Fruity Sparkling
Unflavored	Sugar Alcohols	Water
	Bouillon	Gum
	Store- Made Broth	Breath Mints
	Coffee Creamer	Homemade Bone
	Anything with	Broth
	Calories	Coconut Oil
		Butter
		Heavy Cream

Challenge:

Now that you have been intermittent fasting for several weeks, it is time to challenge yourself. A good way to do this is pick one "Challenge Day" a week and try extending your fast that day. For example, if you follow an 18:6 pattern most days, pick a day and extend your fast to 20-22 hours or eat OMAD that day. This was tough for me at first. I had conquered 18:6 and felt pretty comfortable with that pattern. I decided to throw one challenge day in a week and only eat one meal a day. Just like morning fasting, I found myself hungry every few hours, but if I kept busy when the hunger waves hit, I had no problem holding off eating until dinner. I actually like the days where I only eat OMAD because it frees up so much time and I don't need to worry about meal prep or clean up for most of the day!

When you are first starting to incorporate challenge days, I encourage you to pick a day when you are going to be busy, but not super active. Keeping your mind occupied helps you to not think about food all day. Picking a day when you are not especially physically active can help keep hunger under control. It's not smart to plan a challenge day for when you have an 8-mile training run or a hard exercise class.

If you are already following an OMAD pattern, you could try doing an overnight fast and see how you feel. If you do, add a little sea salt to your water or drink a bit of pickle juice for extra sodium. An Epsom salt bath that evening will help you replenish magnesium and may improve sleep.

Again, think about what your goals are. If your primary goal is weight loss or reversing diabetes, then an overnight fast and even longer fasts can be very helpful. If you are practicing intermittent fasting for other health benefits, then overnight or extended fasts may not be something you want to try.

If you are trying extended fasts past 1 day, add a pinch of sea salt to your water each day for extra sodium, and take an Epsom Salt bath each night. Add 1-1.5 cups of Epsom to your bath water for extra magnesium. This will help you to avoid any headaches or muscle cramping. You could also try electrolyte drops.

Change:

Are you noticing a pattern? Here is another opportunity to take a look at what you are doing and change things up that are not working. I never want you to stay in a pattern too long if you feel unwell or are not making any progress.

Remember the scale may not move as much as you would like when you begin intermittent fasting. I promise you there are other changes going on within your body. You may have a lot of healing to do and your body doesn't want to let go of the weight. If you have been very toxic for a long time, remember toxins are often stored in fat tissue and detox needs to happen little by little. Your body knows best, so trust it.

If you feel well, keep at it, little by little. There are so many benefits to fasting that are not scale related. Notice the changes that are happening in your body composition, sleeping, stress, and overall well-being. These are all important! This is a good time to take measurements again if you haven't already done so. You may be amazed at the mass you have lost! Take another picture and truly look at how far you have come.

Again, look at your overall nutrition and change things up if you need to. Are you still eating processed foods? Are you eating too many carbohydrates? Not enough? Are you eating enough fat? Fiber?

If you are stuck, I encourage you to journal and write down what you are eating. You do not need to track every little thing because that is no fun, but writing down your food intake can help you make connections between mood, and any other symptoms you may be experiencing. Are you getting headaches? Bloating? Feeling blue? Write down what you eat, your sleep and lifestyle habits, and what symptoms you experience. This can help you see what is triggering unwanted symptoms so you can decide how to heal that symptom from within. Lastly, make sure your fasts are clean!

E- EASE Your Mind

Weeks 12 and beyond

Congratulations! You made it through 12 weeks of Nutritional PEACE! I sincerely hope you are feeling better and have learned about your body, nutritional needs and how to feel your best. The last step of Nutritional PEACE does not have a time frame as these are life habits that need to be managed at all times. In particular, we need to look at stress and sleep, and how they relate to your health and well-being.

Stress

We have looked at the hormone cortisol, which is released by your adrenal gland during times of stress. By being continually stressed, cortisol is continually released. Prolonged cortisol stimulation will raise glucose levels, which will raise insulin. This increase in insulin can play a substantial role in weight gain.

Now we know why it is so hard to lose or maintain weight and health under periods of constant stress!

You may know cortisol as "the stress hormone" because it mediates the flight-or-fight response. The fight-or-flight response sets off a whole host of physiological responses when there is a perceived threat. Thousands of years ago, most human threats were physical, and cortisol preps the body to take action by fighting or fleeing. Once released, cortisol enhances the availability of glucose by telling the cells to release it. In Paleolithic times this was necessary to help us run and avoid being eaten. In the distant past, humans typically burned up these releases in energy because physical exertion soon followed the start of the stressful event.

The body is well adapted to short-term increases in cortisol and glucose levels. However, chronic stress causes a big problem, and most stress in today's society is chronic. We are not running from tigers or fighting off predators. We are dealing with work stress, family stress, financial stress, and chronic health issues.

Under conditions of chronic stress, glucose levels remain high, as the perceived stressor is continuous and never dealt with. In many cases of chronic stress, blood glucose may remain high for months, triggering the constant release of insulin. Many studies show increased levels of cortisol increases insulin resistance.

That's not good news for those under chronic stress.

We all have stress in our lives, that is just part of being human. How you deal with it and let it affect you will make a huge difference in whether you develop or resolve chronic health issues. This is where exercise, yoga, massage and meditation can play a key role in resolving chronic stress. Sitting in front of a TV, computer, or having a phone glued to your hand is not a good way to relieve stress! Getting out for a walk after a long day of work where cortisol may have been stimulated multiple times is crucial for burning off that extra glucose released from cells. Go outside, get some exercise, breath fresh air, be in the sun, meditate.

What is your biggest source of stress right now?
How can it be resolved, or at least better managed?
What can you do to keep cortisol levels minimal?

You may need to make some major life changes in order to better manage stress. A job change, a move, severing a toxic relationship... while these are all difficult choices to make, they may be critical to restore and maintain health. Reducing stress is difficult, but in most cases, mandatory. You can implement this entire program, but if your stress is not managed, it can be one step forward and two steps back until you are at a better place with overall stress.

Stress can be physical, chemical or emotional. It is important that all areas are managed. Just one little leak in any area can cause a flat tire! Again, stress is a part of life, but it is important that major life stress is dealt with in order to have longstanding success with weight management and maintaining good health.

Sleep

Sleep is another cause of chronic stress and poor health. Short sleep duration is consistently linked to weight gain. Sleeping only 5-6 hours is associated with a 50% increase in weight gain!

Sleep deprivation also stimulates cortisol. Uh oh, we know what that means! A single night of sleep deprivation increases cortisol levels by more than 100%. By the next evening, cortisol is still 37-45% higher. You can see how constant sleep deprivation leads to chronically elevated cortisol, which leads to elevated glucose, which leads to stimulation of insulin, which leads to weight gain. Sleep deprivation will clearly undermine weight loss and efforts to reduce chronic health issues. Getting enough good sleep (7-8 hours in adults) is essential to any weight loss plan and maintaining good health.

If you don't have good sleep hygiene, it is critical you implement it now. This means making sleep a high priority and creating an atmosphere that induces restful sleep. Go to bed around the same time each night and wake up around the same time each morning, even on weekends. Sleeping in cooler temperatures with very minimal, if any, light is helpful. Avoid looking at your phone or any screens for at least an hour before bed. By now, you are not eating hours before bed, and this will help promote better sleep as well because your body will not have to focus on food digestion. Turning off your Wi-Fi at night can reduce EMF interference, which can induce better sleep as well.

Nutritional PEACE at a Glance

P: Prepare, Weeks 1 and 2

Prepare your body for fasting by eliminating processed and fake foods as much as possible. Plan your meals each week. Avoid foods with GMO's and eat organic food as much as possible. Avoid obesogens. Stop eating at least 3 hours before bedtime and avoid snacking in between meals.

E: Extend Fasts, Weeks 3 and 4

Start with 12-14 hours of fasting, eating with a 10 to 12 hour window. Extend to 16-18 hours of fasting as tolerated. When comfortable with that, extend fasts to 20-22 hours or try OMAD once or twice a week. Break your fast and eat if you feel dizzy or unwell. Feel free to switch it up each day and rotate days of longer eating times and higher carbohydrates. Take it hour by hour!

A: Alter Nutrition, Weeks 5 - 8

This is the time to take a look at your nutritional intake and tweak it as needed. Make sure your meals are balanced, nutrient-dense and varied. Eat with the seasons and try new things! If you are struggling with fasting times, look at your fat intake and increase it if needed. Avoid processed foods during your eating window to make fasting easier.

C: Clean, Challenge and Change, Weeks 9 - 12

Look at your fasting time and make sure it is clean, especially if you are struggling with hunger or stalled weight loss. Challenge yourself by choosing 1 day a week to extend your fast. Try OMAD at least weekly if you haven't done so already. This is a good time to try an extended fast if you are doing well with daily fasting and have a lot of weight to lose or are working on reversing type 2 diabetes. Try a 3 day fast over a 2 day fast, as day 2 tends to be the hardest in terms of appetite, and one you get past that, your appetite will likely diminish significantly. Change things up weekly or monthly to keep your body guessing!

E: Ease Your Mind, Weeks 12 and Beyond

Focus on reducing stress as needed and protecting sleep. These 2 parts of your life are critical in achieving and maintaining optimal health. Pinpoint your biggest stressor(s) and list at least 3 ways you can reduce stress in that area(s) of your life. Keep track of your sleep and aim for at least 7-8 hours of solid sleep each night.

Final Thoughts

The amount of weight loss and overall healing varies tremendously from person to person. One person may lose 8 pounds in 2 weeks and the next loses .8 pounds but is sleeping much more soundly and experiencing more energy.

The longer you have struggled with obesity, the more difficult you may find it to lose weight. Your body has a lot of healing to do and has been insulin resistant for a long, long time. Certain medications may make it more difficult to lose weight and heal. The best advice I can give you is to be patient and persistent. *Don't get overwhelmed or give up.* Take it day by day, hour by hour. Your health will improve!

You will likely experience a plateau at some point, this is normal. As we learned, changing up your fasting routine and/or food intake may stimulate continued weight loss. This may be a good time to change up the times in which you are fasting, or try an extended fast if you haven't already. Changing your fasting protocol may be what is necessary to break through a plateau.

Fasting requires patience and practice, just like any other life skill. Don't give up when you hit a bump in the road! Although it has virtually been a part of human culture dating back as far as we know, many people in Westernized civilizations have never fasted in their lives.

Unfortunately, fasting has been feared and rejected by mainstream nutritional authorities as difficult and even dangerous. Nothing could be further from the truth! The truth, in fact, is the exact opposite. Eating too much of the wrong foods and eating all the time has made us sick and fat as a society.

It's time to change and recover your health. *Your body can and will heal* if given the correct building materials and environment. You now have the tools for success!

I am proud of you for caring enough to read this book, and making choices to improve your health, no matter what the outcome.

PART 5: NUTRITIONAL PEACE SUCCESS STORIES

Laurie H.

Laurie started at a weight of 254 and now weighs 220. She is still actively losing weight and inches! She has lost a total of 23.5 inches and has a lower resting heart rate.

She has been intermittent fasting daily, and primarily follows a keto diet. She implements 3-day fasts at least monthly, and in the beginning, she implemented them weekly.

Here is more about her story that I will keep updating:

Laurie: I have been heavy (chunky was a kind description back then) for most of my life. I had a few years of high school when I was in great shape and not overweight. I gained 60 pounds while pregnant with my son at the end of high school.

I managed to work out 5-6 days a week doing aerobic exercise and some weight lifting and lost about 40 of it around the age of 22. I continued to put on weight over the years and weighed about 165 at the age of 28. I got pregnant again with twins and gained weight again. After I gave birth I was up to 201 when I came home from the hospital.

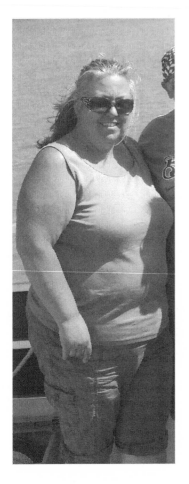
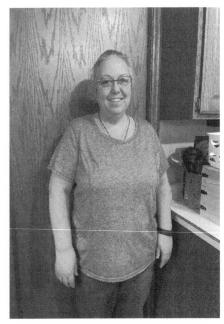

Laurie before and after
implementing Nutritional
PEACE

As a stay at home mom, and with McDonalds just a few blocks
away, convenience foods led to more weight gain. I remember
being 227 in 2010. I have continued to put on weight despite
trying to eat healthy foods and minimizing my sugar intake.

Since 2016, when I turned 50 years old, I have been on a
wellness journey. I have tried many things- supplements, good
fats, cut out soda for a time, walking for exercise, but nothing
helped me keep the weight off. I even did Whole 30 for a month
and lost 13 pounds, but it wasn't long and it returned.

Finally, in October of 2019 I started working with Shana and have had tremendous success! I have learned the truth about WHY I couldn't keep the weight off and that over the years my body metabolically has sort of turned against me! I have had a lot of issues in the past 3 years with my knees, torn meniscuses both with surgery, and it left me unable to get the exercise I had been doing. Then, emergency gallbladder surgery and an umbilical hernia surgery (from the gallbladder surgery), all 4 in just 3 years! UGH. I have dealt with swelling in my feet and a bloated belly after eating. Irritable Bowel Syndrome has plagued me for years!

Joint pain has been an issue for me as well. I learned that our knees carry four times our weight! That is a lot of work for my knees! Another area that I have been struggling with for about the last 3-4 years is a skin rash on my legs. Mostly just on my calves. I imagine this is some sort of allergic reaction, just not sure to what. I was tired all of the time and didn't sleep very well. Losing the weight has definitely improved most of my health issues. There are just a couple that I am trying to figure out yet.

I tried to lose weight by doing the standard calorie counting... calories in lower than calories out. Exercising a ton, to the point of issues with shin splints. Eventually the weight always came back. I tried Whole 30 and lost some weight initially but didn't make it a lifestyle change because it was just too hard to feed my family that way.

Now, my clothes fit a lot better, I had to buy a size smaller pair of jeans and now those are baggy too! Even my shirts are hanging differently. I think the biggest non-scale victory is the emotional change I have. I now know that it isn't all my fault that I couldn't loose weight. Sure, I have a responsibility to make good choices about how much I eat. BUT I feel so much more confident in my choices and the control I have over my body and health! There one non-scale victory that I am excited to see come to fruition! I want to experience flying on an airplane with all of the weight and inches I have lost! I could always buckle the seat belt but there wasn't any "extra slack" on the belt... I anticipate some slack when I fly next!

Any struggles?

One thing I have noticed is some joint pain. I have had this before but I am wondering if there is a connection to being in ketosis with ketones. Another area is the skin rash on my legs. It seems to linger, not sure what foods it coming from, if any. I have noticed that I am a little bit crabbier on my fasting days. I can tell that I am crabby because I am hungry.

Where are you on your health journey?

I think the main thing is my thinking about how much I can control my progress where before I really felt hopeless. I am really enjoying learning how insulin affects our body and our overall health! I am excited to continue learning and discovering the freedom that fasting brings! Instead of years of fearing food!

I feel that in some ways I am just beginning this journey because of the truth being revealed but otherwise I am very motivated and feel encouraged to move to the next level of better health. I used to dream of being a runner! Since my knee surgeries I have let go of that dream! BUT I really want to continue to lose weight and hopefully get under 200 and eventually maybe about 165/170! I am also hoping to help others by being an example of how it's never too late to make some changes to positively impact your health!

Congratulations Laurie! We love your story!

Leslie and John

Leslie: Just after the New Year of 2020, John and I were both at our heaviest weights. We were not feeling great and were struggling with mood, activity level and overall gut health. We decided we had to do something. I (Leslie) had signed up for Shana's *Introduction to Intermittent Fasting* class and John did some research on low carb eating. After the class, we jumped right in!

We are both fasting from about 7:00 pm -11:30 am. We have gone low carb, although we don't follow keto or count carbohydrates. As of the time of this writing (2/27/2020), John has lost 30 pounds and I have lost 17. Our clothes fit substantially better, and we are no longer bloated! We feel better about ourselves and it is influencing our relationship, and our relationship with others, especially in the area of mood.

Shana's class opened my eyes to many things. I replaced in my head the information about what we used to learn about dieting and what we now know. I have increased healthy fats and given myself permission to eat them! I used to have a lot of guilt around this. We are eating cleaner and I do not need as many carbohydrates to fuel my runs. I have had a major shift in thinking and I believe it is what my body has best responded to. There were so many years of running and dieting and not feeling fit. I feel so much better!

Shana, thank you for sharing your knowledge, it is making a big impact on our entire family!

Paige

Age: 16

Main Health Issue: Acne

Strategies Implemented: Decreased sugars and processed foods, intermittent fasting 15-18 hours daily

Like many high school teenagers, Paige started struggling with acne around the age of 13. Her inflamed skin interfered with her self-confidence and caused constant worry. She tried several topical acne cleansers, toners, facemasks, and moisturizers, but these over-the-counter treatments did little to improve the health of her skin.

Rather than disrupting the delicate balance of her skin with a prescribed acne medication, Paige agreed to work with Shana and implemented her recommended strategies.

Within a few weeks her skin began to naturally heal. Paige now feels more confident and enjoys the life of a happy teenager. Her nutrition strategies are flexible, allowing her those occasional splurges and treats.

Paige's main strategies were to decrease sugars and overall processed carbohydrates. She also increased healthy fats in her diet to nourish her skin from within and support hormone balance. She avoids eating after dinner and pushes her breakfast time back to mid-morning most days. This allows her body additional healing time. Paige finds this lifestyle works well for her, as she usually doesn't feel hungry until later in the morning. She does not restrict calorie intake in any way and eats until she feels full during her eating window.

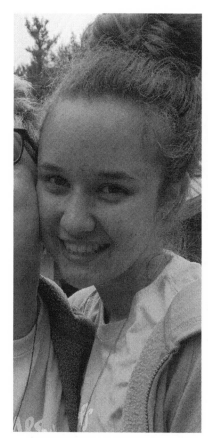

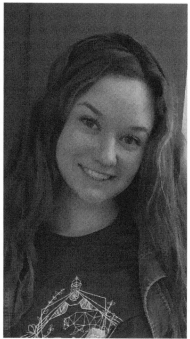

Paige before
and after

Melissa

Melissa has struggled with her weight since early childhood. She remembers being in 4th grade and overhearing older kids talking about how they had finally cracked 100 pounds. She was already over 100 pounds.

Shortly after her 13th birthday, her mom had her thyroid tested, because even though she was restricting her food intake, she was still gaining weight. She was diagnosed with hypothyroidism and was placed on daily medication to manage her thyroid hormones. Her parents left it up to her to take her medication, but she didn't take it regularly until she was in her early 20's.

During the decades of her weight struggles, Melissa tried restricting food intake, limiting fat, and implementing various exercise programs. She enrolled with Weight Watchers several times. With all of these strategies, she would lose weight for a while, but then gain it all back.

In 2004 at her heaviest weight of around 330 pounds, she decided to have gastric bypass surgery. She did lose a large amount of weight but never managed to get below 200 pounds. At that time the aftercare for gastric bypass was not as

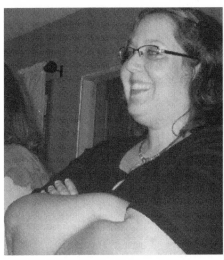
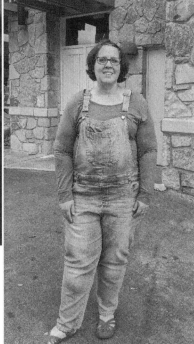

Melissa before and after

thorough as it is now, and Melissa ended up gaining back a lot of the weight that she lost.

As Melissa got older, weight loss became more difficult. Although she has always been fairly confident with good self-esteem she feels her extra weight has aged her. She feels unable to do the things she wants to do with her husband and 6 children. She does not want to feel limited anymore.

In Nov of 2019, she started intermittent fasting and implemented strategies Shana recommended. Since then she has lost 35.5 pounds and is still actively losing. Her hormones are getting back into balance. Although there were some setbacks such as holidays and irregular schedules, she still managed to lose weight.

This is what Melissa had to say:

"This is the best lifestyle change I have ever tried. It's so sustainable. I've gotten loads of comments on my weight loss. My body is changing and I'm down 2 pants sizes. I am much more active than I was just a few short months ago."

Shana, thank you for educating me about this lifestyle and for being so encouraging. The support and not being judged is so wonderful."

Jeni

The 6 months prior to working with Shana, Jeni had been experiencing fatigue, sleep disturbances, acne which she had never had, and bloating. She was starting to gain a few pounds around her middle. She had never experienced weight issues in her life!

Here is more from Jeni:

Truly, I feel like I met my goals AND THEM SOME by day 2! I was already at a healthy weight when starting the program, exercised consistently, drank plenty of water and had a healthy diet and took high-quality vitamins, which worked my whole life until I turned 42 and peri- menopause showed up as insomnia, acne on my neck and jawline, heavy periods, hot flashes and mood swings. Fasting was the "missing link" I needed to work with the good choices I was already making.

Below is a list of immediate improvements I noted:

Chronic inflammation in left side of neck is almost completely gone
More energy
Deeper and more relaxed breathing
Improved mental clarity and alertness
Clear skin
Sleeping much better
No hot flashes at night, actually back to warmer pajamas
Wake up refreshed and not groggy
Less aches/pains
Appreciate food more
Weight is the same, BUT my stomach flat and clothes are looser

I don't remember ever feeling this good!

My long-term goals are to continue fasting, incorporate eating fruit and veggies in season, gradually increase my exposure to the sun to build up my vitamin D stores and to continue working on my sleep, which is already much better.

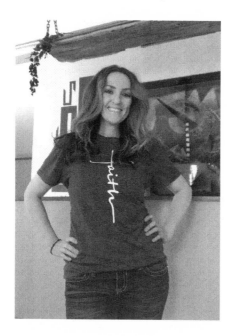

Congratulations, Jeni!

Heather

I have struggled with weight gain/loss, lack of energy, and most importantly constipation issues my entire life. I have been on all kinds of diets since I was 10 years old. I have had many successes along the way, but none of what I tried lasted long-term with longevity.

One thing I did try that helped me not feel bloated and gave me more energy was watching my carbohydrate intake. With all the yo-yo diets, I was learning things about my body along the way, but the one thing that stayed the same was my inability to have regular bowel movements. I would go 2-3 weeks without having a bowel movement. Most of those times, I would need to take some type of a laxative to help the process. I have tried everything under the sun and was really excited about how I was feeling with less carbs in my life, but the scale was not moving like I wanted it to and neither were my bowels.

With the lack of sunlight, the scale not moving, continued constipation, and a little feeling of depression, my husband told me it was time to contact Shana. That was the best decision I could have made. Shana met with me and listened to my story, and through laughter and tears I was able to tell her my frustrations and successes I have had for the past 35 years. She was encouraging and gave me this feeling of hope that I have never felt before.

We met on a Friday and by Monday I was starting a new way of life through intermittent fasting with carb cycling once a week. It has been amazing! The scale is moving in the right direction (10 pounds down in a month), but most importantly, I am having a bowel movement at least 3-5 times a week. This way of life has been a game changer for me.

I now shop around the outside aisles in the grocery store (veggies, fruits, less processed foods), and stopped drinking soda. Having a BM on a regular basis is a feeling that I have never experienced. I was always so jealous of the people in my life that started their day with a good BM. Well, I can finally say that is me most days! Food used to control me and I am starting to feel that role reversal change.

Thank you to Shana and *Fast to Heal* for helping me feel healthy inside and out.

Leanne

Leanne's Mom got in touch with me as Leanne had struggled with long-term ADHD, anxiety, weight issues her entire life, sugar and carbohydrate cravings, and sleep issues. She had also been experiencing digestive issues for at least 5 years.

After she went away for her first year at college, she gained more weight and it was getting increasingly difficult for her to focus on homework and studies. Being a math major, she needed to focus on math problems for hours at times. Her Mom reported to me that she constantly craved processed carbohydrates, and no matter how many she ate, never felt full.

I talked Leanne and her Mom through strategies to try and report back to me how things were going. Within a few days, I got this message:

"Leanne said she can tell this is working. She worked on one Math problem for 3 hours straight and never lost focus. She has never been able to do that before. She is doing really well so far. She lost 4 pounds in the first week and is encouraged to keep going with this lifestyle! She is only eating 6 hours out of the day and takes in about 50 grams of natural carbohydrates. She increased her protein and healthy fats. Focus and ADHD has already improved. She is reading your book and her body is getting used to this lifestyle."

Congratulations, Leanne, I can't wait to see how the rest of your journey unfolds!

I genuinely LOVE hearing all the success stories, and can't wait to hear YOURS! Please submit them to me at any time.

~Shana

A Day in the Life of Shana

I thought it might be helpful for you to see what my typical routine is, what and when I eat, how I structure my day.

I am up pretty early, usually by 6. If my kids have school, I help them get ready for their day. After they leave I typically try and get my exercise in after that- walking, running, hiking or strength training, for about an hour. Then I work or write depending on what I have going. If I am able, I like to do my exercise late in the morning or early in the afternoon. That way, I can break my fast within a few hours of my exercise session.

I love hot tea in the morning when it is cold out. I break my fast somewhere between 12-2 most days. A typical lunch would be a salad or tuna salad with avocado mayo, celery, pickles. I eat a lot of leftovers!

I try not to snack in between meals and we usually eat dinner around 6-6:30. We eat a lot of game meat as my husband hunts a lot. I do eat potatoes often, and lots of vegetables. I eat healthy fats at every meal. I enjoy many hearty soups in the winter and salads in the summer. I love a piece or two of dark chocolate after meals!

I very rarely eat after dinner; it has to be a very special occasion. On the weekends, I tend to have a glass or two of wine before dinner, but not much alcohol other than that, maybe a Bloody Mary on the weekend. I drink a lot of water! I don't knowingly eat gluten and eat few grains, as I feel bloated and uncomfortable if I do.

Pretty ordinary, but hope it's helpful!

Shana

ABOUT THE AUTHOR

Shana Hussin, RDN has worked in the medical nutrition therapy field for 20 years. Like most dietitians, she recommended strategies for her clients for most of her career that didn't work long-term. She grew very frustrated with conventional nutrition approaches and even left the field for several years, serving as a substitute teacher during that time.

Thankfully, she stumbled upon the work of Dr. Jason Fung, MD and developed a weight loss program for her clients that resulted in immediate success. Determined to share the correct information with as many as she could reach, she wrote this step-by-step book.

Shana and her husband have 3 children and live in Kaukauna, WI. When she is not writing or working with clients, she enjoys reading, running, traveling, boating, walking with friends and cheering her children on in whatever they are pursuing.

www.fasttoheal.info
shana@fasttoheal.info

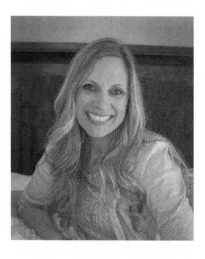

159